Non-Invasive Skin Treatments

Editor

JAMES NEWMAN

FACIAL PLASTIC SURGERY CLINICS OF NORTH AMERICA

www.facialplastic.theclinics.com

Consulting Editor
ANTHONY P. SCLAFANI

November 2023 • Volume 31 • Number 4

ELSEVIER

1600 John F. Kennedy Boulevard • Suite 1800 • Philadelphia, Pennsylvania, 19103-2899

http://www.theclinics.com

FACIAL PLASTIC SURGERY CLINICS OF NORTH AMERICA Volume 31, Number 4
November 2023 ISSN 1064-7406, ISBN-13: 978-0-443-18244-0

Editor: Stacy Eastman
Developmental Editor: Shivank Joshi

Facial Plastic Surgery Clinics of North America (ISSN 1064-7406) is published quarterly by Elsevier Inc., 360 Park Avenue South, New York, NY 10010-1710. Months of issue are February, May, August, and November. Business and Editorial Offices: 1600 John F. Kennedy Blvd., Suite 1800, Philadelphia, PA 19103-2899. Periodicals postage paid at New York, NY, and additional mailing offices. Subscription prices are $428.00 per year (US individuals), $728.00 per year (US institutions), $477.00 per year (Canadian individuals), $904.00 per year (Canadian institutions), $568.00 per year (foreign individuals), $904.00 per year (foreign institutions), $100.00 per year (US students), $100.00 per year (Canadian students), and $255.00 per year (foreign students). Foreign air speed delivery is included in all *Clinics* subscription prices. All prices are subject to change without notice. POSTMASTER: Send address changes to *Facial Plastic Surgery Clinics*, Elsevier Health Sciences Division, Subscription Customer Service, 3251 Riverport Lane, Maryland Heights, MO 63043. **Customer service: 1-800-654-2452 (US and Canada); 1-314-447-8871 (outside US and Canada); Fax: 314-447-8029; E-mail: journalscustomerservice-usa@elsevier.com (for print support); journalsonlinesupport-usa@elsevier.com (for online support).**

Reprints. For copies of 100 or more of articles in this publication, please contact the Commercial Reprints Department, Elsevier Inc., 360 Park Avenue South, New York, NY 10010-1710. Tel.: 212-633-3874; Fax: 212-633-3820; E-mail: reprints@elsevier.com.

Facial Plastic Surgery Clinics of North America is covered in *MEDLINE/PubMed* (*Index Medicus*).

Contributors

CONSULTING EDITOR

ANTHONY P. SCLAFANI, MD, MBA, FACS
Director of Facial Plastic Surgery Professor of
Otolaryngology- Head & Neck Surgery Weill
Cornell Medical College, New York, New York,
USA

EDITOR

JAMES NEWMAN, MD, FACS
Medical Director, Premier Plastic Surgery,
Palo Alto, California, USA

AUTHORS

MACRENE ALEXIADES, MD, PhD
Associate Clinical Professor, Yale School of
Medicine, New Haven, Connecticut, USA;
Dermatology & Laser Surgery Center of
New York, New York, New York,
USA

RICHARD H. BENSIMON, MD
Plastic Surgery, Bensimon Center, Portland,
Oregon, USA

JASON D. BLOOM, MD, FACS
Department of Otorhinolaryngology–Head and
Neck Surgery, University of Pennsylvania,
Bloom Facial Plastic Surgery, Bryn Mawr,
Pennsylvania, USA

JASON BURTON, MA
University of California, Los Angeles, Los
Angeles, California, USA

ANNE CHAPAS, MD
Union Square Laser Dermatology, New York,
New York, USA

MELODYANNE Y. CHENG, MS
David Geffen School of Medicine at UCLA, Los
Angeles, California, USA

SUNEEL CHILUKURI, MD, FAAD, FACMS
Associate Clinical Professor, Baylor College of
Medicine, CEO, Refresh Dermatology,
Houston, Texas, USA

ANYA COSTELOE, DO
Premier Plastic Surgery, Palo Alto, California,
USA; The Maas Clinic, California Pacific
Heights Medical Center

ARMAN DANIELIAN, MD, MS
Department of Head and Neck Surgery, David
Geffen School of Medicine at UCLA, Los
Angeles, California, USA

MARIE DANIELIAN, PharmD
Independent Researcher, Los Angeles,
California, USA

J. KEVIN DUPLECHAIN, MD, FACS
Adjunct Instructor, Division of Facial Plastic
Surgery, Department of Otolaryngology,
Tulane Medical School, Lafayette, Louisiana,
USA

SOLOMIYA GRUSHCHAK, MD
Department of Dermatology, University of
California, Irvine, Irvine, California, USA

PETER S. HAN, MD
Department of Head and Neck Surgery, David Geffen School of Medicine at UCLA, Los Angeles, California, USA

LAUREN HOFFMAN, MD
Union Square Laser Dermatology, New York, New York, USA

RHORIE P.R. KERR, MD, FACS
Department of Head and Neck Surgery, David Geffen School of Medicine at UCLA, Los Angeles, California, USA

VICTOR G. LACOMBE, MD
Double-Board Certified Facial Plastic Surgeon, Owner and Medical Director, Artemedica, Santa Rosa, California, USA

ANNE S. LOWERY, MD
Department of Otorhinolaryngology–Head and Neck Surgery, University of Pennsylvania, Philadelphia, Pennsylvania, USA

COREY MAAS, MD
The Maas Clinic, California Pacific Heights Medical Center, San Francisco, California, USA

LOUISE MCDONALD, MB, BCh, BAO, BSc (Hons)
Department of Dermatology, Ulster Hospital, Belfast, Northern Ireland, United Kingdom

JAMES NEWMAN, MD, FACS
Medical Director, Premier Plastic Surgery, Palo Alto, California, USA

ANGELA NGUYEN, BS
The Maas Clinic, San Francisco, California, USA

ZAKIA RAHMAN, MD, FAAD
Department of Dermatology, Stanford University School of Medicine

EMILY SEDAGHAT, MD
HCA Florida Kendall Hospital Miami, Florida, USA

LINDSEY VOLLER, MD
Department of Dermatology, Stanford University School of Medicine

HANNAH WAIBEL, BS
Southern Methodist University, Private Practice: Miami Dermatology and Laser Institute, Subsection Chief of Dermatology, Baptist Hospital, Miami, Florida, USA; Voluntary Assistant Professor, Dermatology Faculty, Miller School of Medicine, University of Miami

JILL S. WAIBEL, MD
Southern Methodist University, Private Practice: Miami Dermatology and Laser Institute, Baptist Hospital, Miami, Florida USA; Dermatology Faculty, Miller School of Medicine, University of Miami

ANNI WONG, MD
Department of Otorhinolaryngology–Head and Neck Surgery, University of Pennsylvania, Philadelphia, Pennsylvania, USA

CAMERON M. B. ZACHARY, MD
Department of Dermatology, University of California Irvine, Irvine, California, USA

Contents

Skin Anatomy and Analysis 433

Cameron M.B. Zachary, Solomiya Grushchak, and James Newman

> This article provides a comprehensive review and strong reference for facial and neck anatomy. An anatomic foundation is built for the dermatologic concepts, techniques, procedures, and surgeries detailed in noninvasive skin treatments. Superficial anatomic landmarks have been established that allow for more nuanced navigation and measurement of facial features. Throughout this article, we discuss key anatomic features of the face and neck, compare dermal thickness in various regions and ethnic anatomic differences, review insertion points of retaining ligaments of the superficial musculoaponeurotic system, and detail diagnostic tools including ultrasound and optical coherence tomography analysis of the skin.

Translational Biochemistry of the Skin 443

Lindsey Voller and Zakia Rahman

> Understanding translational biochemistry of the skin is an essential component in mastering non-invasive aesthetic treatments. Collagen is the most abundant protein in the animal kingdom and plays a significant role in maintaining structural function in biologically healthy human skin. Collagen degradation and synthesis occurs throughout human life. Upregulation of collagen synthesis remains the mainstay of non-invasive aesthetic skin treatments. Elastin is a smaller yet significant component in the skin's ability to maintain biologically healthy stretch and recoil. Multi-Omics represents a relatively nascent field in the optimization and development of therapies aimed at the aesthetic improvement of the skin.

Scar Therapy of Skin 453

Jill S. Waibel, Hannah Waibel, and Emily Sedaghat

 Video content accompanies this article at http://www.facialplastic.theclinics.com.

> Scar therapy is truly important in medicine. Patients experience great loss in quality of life with scars. There are many treatment modalities that help treat scars, including topical, intralesional, surgical, and energy-based devices. In addition, early intervention can help mitigate scar formation. Lasers represent a major innovation in the treatment of all types of scars. Treating scars is a multimodal and multispecialty endeavor. This article highlights the use of many therapies to treat scars and scar symptoms including pruritus, pain, and range of motion. This also highlights key literature including multiple recent consensus guidelines in treating scars.

Laser skin rejuvenation was introduced in the mid-1990s. Early ablative laser devices relied on scanner technology that provided significant ablation and longer time on tissue treatments. These early treatments provided significant improvement in the appearance of the skin, but because of the longer treatment times and in some cases excessive treatment, complications such as scarring and hypopigmentation were significant. More recent advances in skin resurfacing technology have now minimized these risks providing certain key principles are observed. These parameters are reviewed in detail to improve the reader's ability to propose and execute proper skin resurfacing treatments.

Facial resurfacing is a fundamental part of rejuvenation but it is often ignored because of the perceived difficulty. Lasers are an option, but they have proved inadequate for difficult rhytids (ie, perioral) both in quality and longevity. Croton oil peels can give excellent results with remarkable permanence. The misconception of danger and difficulty will be dispelled and the reality that these peels can be done in a controlled fashion and are within the grasp of any practitioner will be discussed.

Radiofrequency microneedling is a technique that allows energy to be delivered to specified target depths in the skin via needle electrodes and measures temperature and impedance within the tissue. This method of delivery and real-time feedback has increased safety and efficacy, providing clinically significant improvements in skin laxity, rhytids, and cellulite.

Ultrasound energy is delivered to the dermal and subdermal tissue to induce thermal injury, leading to collagen remodeling and resulting in lifting and tightening of the skin. Ulthera and Sofwave are two Food and Drug Administration-approved systems that have demonstrated clinically significant results in providing eyebrow, submental, and neck lift and minimizing facial fine lines and wrinkles. Patient selection and management of expectations are important components to a successful treatment process. Both devices boast high patient satisfaction rates, minimal recovery time, and excellent safety profile. Ultrasound technology is an effective, nonsurgical option for facial rejuvenation.

Neurotoxins are the most popular nonsurgical aesthetic procedure for men and women of all ages. Five botulinum toxin A (BoNTA) products represent the current palette of available BoNTA for cosmetic use. Off-label uses of BoNTA continue to expand and are now used for skin rejuvenation, to treat various skin disorders, and in facial nerve paralysis. Dermal and subdermal injections of dilute BoNTA has grown in popularity and been shown to improve skin texture and quality.

Common targets for chemodenervation in facial nerve synkinesis are ipsilateral orbicularis oculi, mentalis, depressor anguli oris, buccinator, corrugator muscles, and the ipsilateral and/or contralateral frontalis.

The normal processes of aging in the face are accompanied by facial volume loss. Aesthetic treatments have been developed to restore lost volume to and below the skin. Understanding the properties and appropriate usages of those volumizing fillers is vital to achieving the best outcomes for patients. Gel firmness, cohesivity, hydrophilicity, tissue integration, and collagen stimulatory properties are attributes to take into consideration when deciding on a volumizing filler. Beyond filler properties, a clinician's understanding of facial harmony and natural aging changes help in understanding how to visualize a holistic response to the use of fillers for youthful restoration.

Deoxycholate (deoxycholic acid) and collagenase are naturally occurring substances whose ability to degrade adipose tissue and collagen respectively has given rise to a variety of therapeutic applications. This article will discuss the indications for the use of deoxycholic acid, primarily its well-established role in the non-surgical reduction of submental fat, with a focus on patient assessment, procedural technique, risks, pitfalls, and key clinical tips. It will also review the indications for collagenase as a degradation therapy, its mechanism of action, and benefits in the management of wound healing, scarring, and adipose tissue modification.

Topical defensins have recently gained attention as agents to improve skin composition. This study aimed to aggregate and synthesize studies in the literature assessing the effects of topical defensins on skin composition in the context of its ability to combat signs of aging.

Understanding facial anatomy is a key aspect for successful treatment of age-related changes manifested to facial tissues. Namely, changes to the facial muscles and their connective tissue framework result in an increased soft tissue laxity, leading to wrinkling, sagging, and altered texture. This review elaborates on the use of novel high intensity focused electrical stimulation (HIFES) and Synchronized RF technology to improve facial muscle tone and skin structure, focusing on the technology background and clinical aspects.

Non-surgical services are an important part of many facial plastic surgery practices and can improve patient satisfaction as well as bring new patients to the practice. An aesthetician can help to prepare patients for surgery and non-surgical procedures as well as optimize skin care during the recovery period. The scope of practice of aestheticians varies widely between states. Facial plastic surgeons who are delegating procedures to an aesthetician need to be familiar and comply with the state regulations and be up to date on ongoing changes. The connection between nutrition, skin, aging, and recovery from surgical procedures is a current topic of interest. Multiple studies suggest that nutraceuticals can provide clinically significant benefits for skin, wound healing, and hair.

FACIAL PLASTIC SURGERY CLINICS OF NORTH AMERICA

THE CLINICS ARE AVAILABLE ONLINE!
Access your subscription at:
www.theclinics.com

Foreword

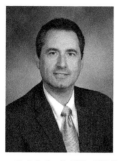

Anthony P. Sclafani, MD, MBA, FACS
Consulting Editor

I am as much interested in the smallest detail as in the whole structure.
—*Marcel Breuer (Architect/designer)*

The skin, the largest organ of the body, is easy to overlook and relegate to a lesser place in the facial plastic surgeon's assessment of the patient. However, it is the skin that the eye's first glance strikes. We notice highlights and shape, as well as blemishes, lines and folds. We also assess the skin for places to hide the evidence of our other procedures, but we debase our results if the skin/soft tissue envelope is not considered.

Early procedures for skin rejuvenation often were accompanied by lengthy recoveries or unwanted sequelae, and we should seek the ideal skin treatment to complement the excellent results achievable with surgical facial rejuvenative treatments. Like skilled architects, Guest Editor James Newman, MD and his authors describe treatment of the facial skin, muscles, and soft tissues as a coherent structure; starting with an assessment of skin anatomy and understanding of the basic qualities of the skin, they expound on minimally invasive treatments to maintain and improve the appearance and quality of the facial skin and soft tissues. These experts review state-of-the-art methods to enhance the appearance of the skin-soft tissue envelope. They focus on this oft-neglected, but most immediately seen, layer. It is when we pay heed to all of our patients' experiences and needs that as clinicians we excel.

God is in the details.
—*Ludwig Mies van der Rohe (Architect)*

Anthony P. Sclafani, MD, MBA, FACS
Department of Otolaryngology
Weill Cornell Medicine
Weill Greenberg Center
1305 York Avenue, Suite Y-5
New York, NY 10021, USA

E-mail address:
ans9243@med.cornell.edu

Facial Plast Surg Clin N Am 31 (2023) xi
https://doi.org/10.1016/j.fsc.2023.06.011
1064-7406/23/© 2023 Published by Elsevier Inc.

Preface
Sign of the Times

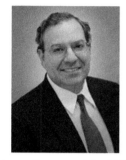

James Newman, MD, FACS
Editor

For the past 10 years, the increasing trend of noninvasive therapies over traditional Facial Plastic Surgery has impacted all of our practices not only because of the patients' desires for minimal downtime but also because of the increasing effectiveness of these therapies, which can complement and enhance our surgical results. For many of us in mature practices, we have seen the average age of patients seeking face-lift surgery becoming older as many people are undergoing volume enhancement, energy-based skin treatments, and sophisticated skin care at younger ages for "prejuvenation" prior to considering surgery. In this issue, we review some of the most important advances in noninvasive treatments from experts in our field as well as our Dermatology colleagues. I want to thank our expert contributors, who have given freely of their time in giving the reader an exceptional update with practical details that can be put into practice without delay.

James Newman, MD, FACS
Premier Plastic Surgery
1795 El Camino Real, Suite 200
Palo Alto, CA 94306, USA

E-mail address:
newman_md@hotmail.com

Facial Plast Surg Clin N Am 31 (2023) xiii
https://doi.org/10.1016/j.fsc.2023.06.001
1064-7406/23/© 2023 Published by Elsevier Inc.

Skin Anatomy and Analysis

Cameron M.B. Zachary, MD[a], Solomiya Grushchak, MD[a],*,
James Newman, MD[b]

KEYWORDS

• Anatomy • Skin • Analysis • Face • Neck

KEY POINTS

• Comprehensive review of skin anatomy of the face and neck.
• Dermal thickness of face and neck in various regions.
• Compare ethnic anatomic characteristics.
• Insertion points of retaining ligaments of the SMAS.
• Ultrasound and OCT analysis of the skin.

ANATOMIC REGIONS AND LANDMARKS OF THE FACE AND NECK

The surface of the face is divided into cosmetic or aesthetic units outlined by the predictable contours of the face.[1,2] The cosmetic units of the face include the forehead, temple, cheeks, nose, periorbital region, lips, and chin, each of which are further divided into smaller subunits. Typically, the skin in each unit is consistent in color, texture, thickness, and mobility.[2] The anatomic regions of the face are indicated in **Fig. 1**A.

Through the study of cephalometry, superficial anatomic landmarks have been established that allow for more nuanced navigation and measurement of facial features.[3] A sound understanding of this nomenclature provides a useful map for the procedural approaches and techniques discussed in this article, and highlights regions that require care and caution to explore and manipulate. The major facial landmarks are indicated in **Fig. 1**B.

In the neck, important landmarks include the hyoid bone, thyroid cartilage, and sternocleidomastoid muscles.

FACE AND NECK MUSCULATURE

The muscles of the face are general divided into two groups: muscles of facial expression and muscles of mastication. Muscles of facial expression (ie,

mimetic muscles) contract the skin of the face and act as sphincters for the eyes, nose, and mouth. These are thin, flat muscles innervated by the facial nerve. The mimetic muscles tend to blend into one another on dissection and there is variability in facial muscles among individuals. The muscles of mastication include the masseter, temporalis, and pterygoid muscles, with the former two being the most relevant in facial surgery (**Fig. 2**).[2]

Important muscles of the neck include the sternocleidomastoids and platysma. The sternocleidomastoid muscle arises by two heads: the sternal head originating on the superior portion of the sternum, and the clavicular head, originating on the medial third of the clavicle. The muscles insert on the outer surface of the mastoid process and the lateral one third of the superior nuchal line. These important anatomical landmarks separate the neck into anterior and posterior triangles. Of the two, the posterior triangle of the neck is of most significance, as the spinal accessory (11th cranial nerve) rests here. The platysma muscle is wide and thin, overlying the sternocleidomastoid muscles. It originates from the superficial fascia of the upper chest and travels over the neck and the border of the jaw to insert at the lateral angle of the mouth. The platysma is a highly variable muscle that is thick and well developed in some individuals, while thin, wispy, and even nonexistent

[a] Department of Dermatology, University of California Irvine, 118 Med Surg 1, Building 810, Irvine, CA 92697, USA; [b] Premier Plastic Surgery, 1795 El Camino Real, Suite 200, Palo Alto, CA 94306, USA
* Corresponding author.
E-mail address: sgrushch@hs.uci.edu

Facial Plast Surg Clin N Am 31 (2023) 433–442
https://doi.org/10.1016/j.fsc.2023.05.004
1064-7406/23/Published by Elsevier Inc.

Abbreviations	
OCT	Optical coherence tomography
SMAS	Superficial musculoaponeurotic system

in others. The muscle is continuous superiorly and laterally with the superficial muscularaponeurotic system (SMAS) of the midface.

FACE AND NECK VASCULATURE

The primary distributing vessels course close to the underlying bony skeleton and emerge from the deep tissues at two specific points: skeletal foramina or where the deep fascia approaches the underlying bone. Most skin and subcutaneous tissue of the face is supplied by the external carotid artery. An exception to this rule is the region of the central face that includes the periorbital area, the upper two-thirds of the nose, and central forehead. These regions are supplied by the ophthalmic branch of the internal carotid artery; however, this system does anastomose with the facial and superficial temporal branches of the external carotid (**Fig. 3**).

RELAXED SKIN TENSION LINES

Relaxed skin tension lines (RSTL) are the lines of skin tension present when the skin is in a relaxed state.[2] In most cases, RSTL follow parallel to wrinkles of the face, but remain distinct entities. Wrinkles and creases become more prominent with age, sun exposure, and continued contraction of facial muscles necessary for facial expression.

Contraction of underlying muscle leads to compression of overlying skin, contributing to prominent wrinkles and creases. Therefore, wrinkles, and commonly RSTL, run perpendicular to the muscle fibers of the face.[1]

However, not all RSTL run parallel to wrinkles. Relatively strong muscle activity in the glabella and temple regions create skin creases nonparallel to RSTLs. These exceptions tend to be surgically insignificant. For example, incisions in the glabellar skin crease heal well.[2] Understanding positioning of RSTLs on the face is crucial for optimal cosmetic and functional repair of surgical defects. Prior studies have revealed closing a wound perpendicular to RSTL requires twice as much tension when compared with a closure designed parallel to RSTL.[4]

LAYERS OF THE FACE

From superficial to deep, the layers of the face consist of five general planes: (1) skin, (2) subcutaneous tissue/superficial areolar tissue, (3) superficial fascia/musculoaponeurotic layer, (4) deep areolar tissue/soft tissue spaces, and (5) periosteum/deep fascia.[5,6]

The relative relationship between these layers is consistent; however, the names of these layers can vary depending on the anatomic region of the face.[5] For example, the superficial fascial layer (layer three) in the mid to lower face is denoted the superficial musculoaponeurotic system (SMAS), whereas the superficial fascial layer in the temporal region superior to the zygomatic arch is denoted by the superficial temporal fascia or temporoparietal fascia.[5] Of note, the term SMAS is

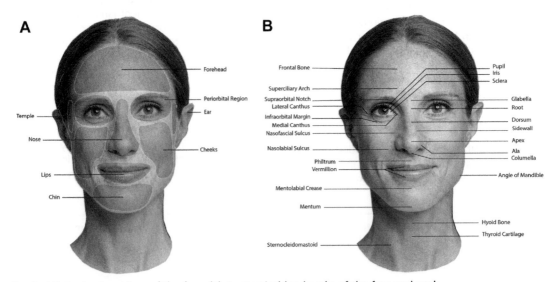

Fig. 1. (*A*) Anatomic regions of the face. (*B*) Anatomical landmarks of the face and neck.

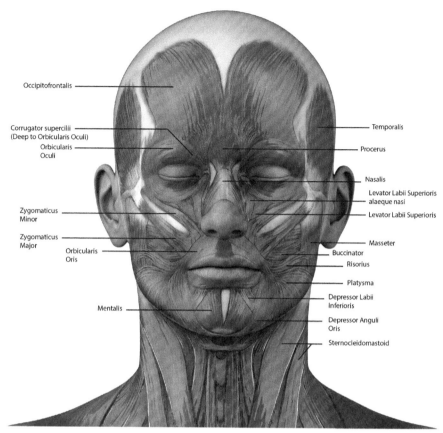

Fig. 2. Superficial muscles of the face and neck.

Occipitofrontalis

Corrugator supercilii
(Deep to Orbicularis Oculi)
Orbicularis
Oculi

Zygomaticus
Minor

Zygomaticus
Major
Orbicularis
Oris

Mentalis

Temporalis

Procerus

Nasalis

Levator Labii Superioris
alaeque nasi

Levator Labii Superioris

Masseter

Buccinator

Risorius

Platysma

Depressor Labii
Inferioris

Depressor Anguli
Oris

Sternocleidomastoid

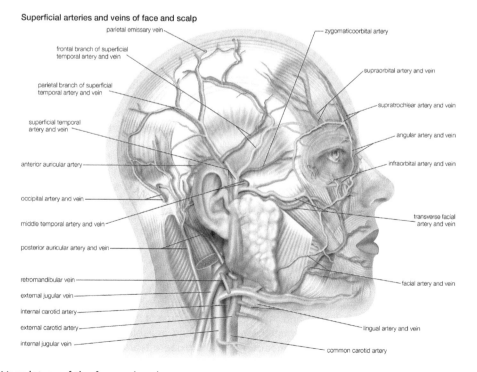

Superficial arteries and veins of face and scalp

parietal emissary vein

frontal branch of superficial
temporal artery and vein

parietal branch of superficial
temporal artery and vein

superficial temporal
artery and vein

anterior auricular artery

occipital artery and vein

middle temporal artery and vein

posterior auricular artery and vein

retromandibular vein

external jugular vein

internal carotid artery

external carotid artery

internal jugular vein

zygomaticoorbital artery

supraorbital artery and vein

supratrochlear artery and vein

angular artery and vein

infraorbital artery and vein

transverse facial
artery and vein

facial artery and vein

lingual artery and vein

common carotid artery

Fig. 3. Vasculature of the face and neck.

broadly used as a proxy term for the superficial fascial layer of the mid to lower face. It is more specifically a complex apparatus including superficial fascia (layer three) and fibrous septae that interlink the skin above with the muscles of facial expression located within layer three. Further information of the SMAS is discussed later.

Throughout the face and neck, the skin varies in thickness, pigmentation, skin appendages, and subcutaneous adherence.[5,7] The skin (layer one) is divided into the thinner, more superficial epidermis and the deeper more fibrous dermis. The greatest total facial skin thickness is the lower nasal sidewall and the thinnest is the upper medial eyelid.[8]

The subcutaneous layer (layer two) contains lobules of fat that are highly vascularized and divided by fibrous septa. The superficial fat compartments (ie, superficial fat pads) are located in the second layer; this subcutaneous fat provides volume for the contours of the face. Visualization of these compartments is achieved via diffusion of injected dye, which stays localized to its respective compartments by boundaries created by septal partitions that originate from the retaining ligaments of the face.[9] Fibrous septa bind the overlying dermis with the underlying superficial fascia layer; they are an integral component of the SMAS located in the mid to lower face.[5,6] The septa that span the subcutaneous layer to the dermis is referred to as the retinacular cutis, which is the most superficial and distal component of the thicker and deeper retaining ligaments that originate from the periosteum or deep fascia in the fifth layer.[6] The retaining ligaments of the face appear in three morphologic forms: adhesions, septa, and true ligaments.[6]

A helpful analogy for understanding the structure and orientation of retaining ligaments and septa is to visualize a tree growing from the periosteum. It's strong roots and trunk make up the deep retaining ligament, and if one follows the trunk through the layers, one eventaully arrives at the skin where the top of the tree lies, where septa are the branches we call the retinacular cutis. Some septa are more *vertically* in line with the deeper retaining ligament, whereas others have branched more *horizonatally,* not overlying the deeper retaining ligament. The density, length, thickness, and orientation of retinacular cutis septa vary depending on the anatomic location on the face and neck. Scalp subcutaneous layer thickness is uniform, thus septa length and reticular cutis fixation is consistent. In contrast the face has varying differences of subcutaneous thickness and dermal attachment. For example, in the nasolabial region, a region with a thick subcutaneous layer, the retinacular cutis septa are long and thus subject to weakening, distention and laxity with age.[6] Conversely in specialized areas, such as the eyelids and lips, the subcutaneous layer is significantly thinner, thus septa running through the layer are shorter and theoretically less prone to deterioration with time.[6] Additionally, reticular cutis septa that are centrally overlying and linearly in line with the deeper retaining ligament are functionally stronger than more horizontally oriented septa on the periphery. Surgically raising subcutaneous flaps where septa are more densely arranged and vertically oriented over underlying retaining ligaments may require a sharp release. Blunt dissection is preferable in subcutaneous compartments not overlying retaining ligaments where septa are less dense and more horizontally oriented.[6]

Deep to the subcutaneous layer lies the superficial fascial layer (layer three). This layer is continuous over the entire face but has unique names depending on the anatomic location.[6] The layer is denoted by the galea aponeurotica over the scalp, the superficial temporal (temporoparietal) fascia over the temples, the orbicularis fascia in the periorbital region, and SMAS over the mid to lower face.[6] The SMAS is contiguous with the platysma in the neck. The SMAS is of particular importance given its wide anatomic surface area, surgical importance, and functional significance for facial expressions.

As described by Larrabee and Makielski,[2] the SMAS is a continuous fibromuscular layer investing and interlinking the muscles of facial expression. The term "musculoaponeurotic" was originally coined because of occasional muscle fibers seen within the superficial fascia over the parotids.[2] The primary component of the SMAS is superficial fascia. The superficial fascia is connected to a meshwork of superficial septa that divide the subcutaneous layer above and ultimately attach to the dermis. The superficial fascial layer also envelops mimetic muscles (muscles of facial expression) in a fibrous sheath. This entire superficial facial apparatus is referred to as the SMAS, which helps transmit, distribute, and amplify facial muscle contractile force to the skin above.

The superficial fascial layer also has thicker durable connections to the deep fascial layer below. These deeper connections provide conduits/protection for branches of nerves and/or arterial blood supply. Some of these connections are particularly dense and are referred to as retaining ligaments that provide integral anchorage and suspension points.[5,7] Examples include the zygomatic ligament and orbicularis retaining ligament.

The fourth layer contains multiple important structures including soft tissue spaces, retaining ligaments, facial nerve branches, and intrinsic muscles that originate from more superficial soft tissue and insert into deeper skeletal attachments.[6] Of note, this layer is where dissection is performed for sub-SMAS facelifts.[6] Soft tissue spaces exist to allow independent movement of periorbital and perioral muscles (located in the roof of the soft tissue space/superficial facial layer) over the major muscles of mastication (located beneath the floor of the soft tissue space/deep fascia layer). Retaining ligaments are found within the boundaries of these soft tissue spaces in the anterior face. In contrast, the lateral region of the face (ie, immediately in front of the ear, extending 2.4–3 cm anterior of the ear cartilage down to the posterior border of the platysma) contains a region of diffuse ligamentous attachment, referred to as the platysma auricular fascia.[6] No mimetic muscles are observed in this region, therefore no soft tissue spaces are present. Here, the dermis, subcutaneous layer, superficial fascia, and underlying parotid capsule are bound together, resulting in a region with a high density of retaining ligaments.[6]

The fifth and final soft tissue layer of the face is the deep fascial layer and periosteum. Similar to the superficial fascial layer, this plane has varying names contingent on anatomic locations and the structures it overlies. When overlying bone, it is referred to as the periosteum. When overlying the muscles of mastication (ie, temporalis and masseter muscles), the deep fascia is the fascial covering of these muscles, denoted as the deep temporal fascia and the masseteric fascia above and below the zygomatic arch, respectively.[6] Overlying the parotid glands the layer is denoted the parotid fascia. The deep fat compartments (also known as preperiosteal fat) are also located in layer five.[6,9]

FAT COMPARTMENTS

Within the face exist two broad categories of fat compartments: superficial and deep. The size, thickness, and density of fat pads vary depending on location.[7] The superficial fat pads are located in the second layer and extend from the nasolabial fold medially to the preauricular and lateral cheek regions laterally. From medial to lateral, these pads are subdivided into the nasolabial fat, superficial medial cheek, middle cheek, and lateral temporal fat compartments.[7,10] The infraorbital fat lies directly superior to the superficial medial cheek, and the infraorbital fat, superficial medial cheek, and nasolabial fat are collectively known as the "malar fat" of the midface.[7]

Just below the superficial fat pads exist the deep fat pads generally located within the deep facial / periosteum layer (layer five). Within the superior midface, deep fat compartments cover the maxilla and zygomatic bones bilaterally, providing contour and volume to the face. The deep fat compartments include the medial and lateral suborbicularis oculi compartments (SOOF), deep medial cheek (divided into a medial and lateral components), and the buccal fat pad.[7,10]

Imaging and histologic studies have revealed contrasting behaviors in growth between superficial and deep fat pads with aging.[10–12] Although it is unclear what influences these changes, superficial fat pads have been observed to hypertrophy with age, whereas deep fat compartments are more likely to atrophy (**Fig. 4**).[11,12]

RETAINING LIGAMENTS OF THE SUPERFICIAL MUSCULOAPONEUROTIC SYSTEM AND SOFT TISSUE SPACES

As previously described, the fourth layer of the face contains natural soft tissue spaces. These spaces are bordered by retaining ligaments whose function is to strategically anchor the soft tissue of the face to the deep fascia or skeletal structures beneath. The roof and floor of these spaces are the third and fifth layers, respectively, and the walls of the spaces are the retaining ligaments. These ligaments also act as conduits for vasculature and branches of the facial nerve. Soft tissue spaces are thus surgically important because they provide "safe zones" for dissections, because no structures cross within the spaces and the facial nerve branches are protected within the surrounding retaining ligaments.[6]

The temple regions contain a large soft tissue space that is generally organized into two sections: the upper temporal space (a true soft tissue space) and the lower compartment (not a soft tissue space, but home to surgically important anatomy). These spaces are positioned between the superficial temporal fascia, above, and the deep temporal fascia, below. The space overlies the temporalis muscle whose function is to facilitate movement at the temporomandibular joint and the act of mastication. These upper and lower compartments are divided by the obliquely oriented bilaminar inferior temporal septum. There are no structures within the upper temporal space. Inferior and parallel to the inferior temporal septum is where the temporal branches of the facial nerve travels, just deep to the superficial temporal fascia. The superior temporal septum that divides the upper temple and the forehead, runs parallel to the lateral (deep) branch of the supraorbital nerve.

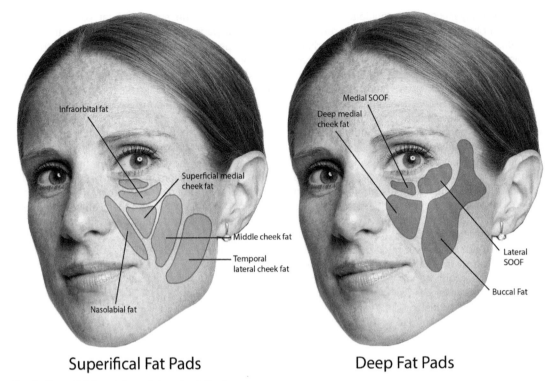

Superifical Fat Pads   Deep Fat Pads

Fig. 4. Superficial and deep fat pads of the face.

Additional important anatomy in this area include the branches of the zygomatic temporal nerve (derived from the zygomatic branch of the maxillary nerve; CN2) and the sentinel vein that is found inferomedial to the inferior temporal septum near the orbital rim.

The prezygomatic space is a triangular-shaped soft tissue space that overlies the body of the zygoma. The roof of this space is the SOOF and overlying orbicularis oculi muscle. The floor is the preperiosteal fat and deeper origins of the zygomatic muscles. The orbicularis retaining ligament makes up the superior boarder of this space, where the sturdier zygomatic ligament makes up the inferior boarder.

Medial to the prezygomatic space, lies the premaxillary space. This space allows for the orbicularis oculi in the roof of the space to move independently from the deeper lip elevator muscles underneath the floor.[6]

The lower premasseter space overlies the inferior half of the masseter. The roof of the space is formed by the platysma. The floor is composed of deep fascia of the masseter. The posterior border is defined as the anterior edge of the parotid gland, and the anterior border is created by the masseteric ligaments near the anterior edge of the masseter. The inferior border is mobile, mesentery-like, and without any ligamentous attachments.[6] Of note,

branches of the marginal mandibular nerve travel along and outside the lower premasseter space; however, no branches travel through the space.

Superior to the lower premasseter space lies the middle premasseter space. The SMAS creates the roof of this space (as opposed to the platysma in the lower premasseter space) and the masseteric fascia forms the floor. Along the superior boarder of the space lies the parotid gland and duct. The upper and lower buccal trunks of the facial nerve are located immediately outside this space along its superior and inferior borders, respectively, making this an ideal safe zone for dissections. The only contents of the space include a portion of the buccal fat pad, which varies per individual.

The buccal space is a potential space located between the overlying platysma and deep facia of the buccinator muscle below. The buccal space is deeper to the previously mentioned spaces. It is situated in the anterior face, just deep to the anterior border of the masseter and above the level of the oral commissure (level depresses below oral commissure with age).[6] The space mostly contains the buccal fat (a deep fat pad), but also contains the parotid duct, minor salivary glands, facial artery and its branches, lymphatic channels, and branches of the facial nerve and mandibular division of the trigeminal nerve.

The soft tissue areas along the perimeter of the orbital and oral cavity do not have the general five-tissue layered anatomy previously discussed. Only the first three layers are present, where the third layer (superficial fascia layer) envelopes the sphincter-like orbicularis muscles (orbicularis oris, orbicularis oculi) that circumferentially line the perimeter of these cavities. Retaining ligaments are condensed and compressed along the borders of these cavities. The inferior medial portion of the periorbital ligament transitions into the orbicularis retaining ligament, which stabilizes the orbicularis oculi muscle to the orbital rim periosteum.[6] Around the mouth, the retaining ligaments arise from the body of the zygoma and from the deep fascia over the masseter.[6]

FACIAL NERVE

The muscles of the face and platysma are all supplied by the facial nerve. The facial nerve is divided into five main branches: (1) frontal (temporal), (2) zygomatic, (3) buccal, (4) marginal mandibular, and (5) cervical rami. The zygomatic and buccal branches tend to have multiple anastomoses between them, in contrast to the temporal and marginal mandibular nerve, which tend to have terminal end points; thus injury to these nerves more often results in ipsilateral paralysis. On the lateral borders of the face, the facial nerve branches exit from the parotid gland below the fifth layer. As these branches travel toward the anterior face, they begin to rise through the fourth layer and ultimately end on the undersurface of the third layer, innervating the mimetic muscles of the musculoaponeurotic layer. These transition points predictably occur at retaining ligaments, which provide stability for the soft tissue structures of the face and protection for nerves. Caution should be used when surgically releasing or manipulating these ligaments.

From a surface view, the temporal branch travels the distance between the tragus and lateral brow. An imaginary line can be constructed between these points, referred to as Pitanguy line. Classically the teaching has been that the temporal branch quickly emerges superficially to just under the SMAS as it passes over the zygomatic arch, thus dissection within this region has been discouraged. However, studies have confirmed that the branches are deeper than previously realized, and rise to the superficial fascia (tempoparietal fascia, layer three) 1.5 to 3 cm above the zygomatic arch.[13,14] Additionally, as the branch courses through the fourth layer, just above the temporalis fascia and periosteum below (fifth layer), it is protected by a separate deep fascial fatty layer named the parotid-temporal fascia (an upward projection of the parotid-masseteric fascia).[13] Results from this study support evidence that specific surgical techniques can safely mobilize the SMAS above the arch, as seen in high-SMAS face lifts.

The zygomatic branch exits the parotid gland deep to the deep fascia just inferior to the zygoma and superior to the parotid duct. The nerve then courses horizontally on top of the masseter along with the transverse facial artery toward the zygomatic ligament and zygomaticus major muscle. The zygomatic ligament (McGregor patch) is a series of retaining ligaments that originates from the periosteum at the junction between the zygomatic arch and zygomatic body. The zygomatic major muscle inserts just medially to the zygomatic ligament. The main zygomatic nerve travels underneath this muscle, supplying the zygomaticus major and minor from beneath. Of note, at the lateral border of the zygomatic ligament, a small motor branch diverges to supply the orbicularis oculi, entering the muscle at its inferolateral border.

As previously discussed, the upper and lower branches of the buccal trunk exit the parotid beneath the level of the masseter fascia and travel along the superior and inferior borders of the mid-premasseter space, respectively. The upper buccal trunk initially travels parallel and superficial to the parotid duct, until it reaches the anterior edge of the masseter where it rises with close association to the upper mesenteric ligament. The lower buccal trunk exits at a more inferior portion of the parotid and travels just under the floor of the superior portion of the lower premasseter space, eventually coursing along the inferior border of the middle premasseter space. Similar to the upper buccal branch, the lower branch rises superficially along the lower mesenteric ligaments to access the underside of the SMAS, eventually innervating the local mimetic muscles of the anterior midface. Of note, as the upper and lower buccal branches reach the third layer, they create anastomoses with one another and other diverging nerves of the zygomatic branches (in addition to the marginal mandibular branches), before innervating the distal mimetic muscles. Therefore, there is much overlap in muscles innervated by these nerves.

The marginal mandibular branch arises from the inferior border of the parotid gland and travels along the inferior border of the mandible. The facial artery is an important landmark that is useful in locating the nerve during surgical procedures. The nerve is always above the inferior border of the mandible while anterior to the facial artery;

however, the position of the branch is variable when posterior to the facial artery.[15] A study revealed that posterior to the facial artery, the branch was along the inferior border of the mandible in 52% of cases, and below the inferior border in 32% of the cases. In the same study, the branch was seen superficial to the facial artery and anterior facial vein in 100% of cases.[15] Of note, anastomosis between the marginal mandibular branch of the facial nerve with other branches of the facial nerve is rare, and explains how transection of this branch typically results in permanent paralysis of the lower lip of that side.

The final division of the facial nerve, the cervical branch, innervates the platysma muscle located along the anterior surface of the neck. A reliable method used to locate the superficial anatomical location of the cervical branch involves creating an imaginary line between the mentum (chin) and mastoid process and then creating another imaginary line that projects perpendicularly from mentum-mastoid line to the angle of the mandible. The cervical branch can be found inferiorly within 1 cm of this intersection.[16]

ETHNIC ANATOMIC CHARACTERISTICS

Gray's anatomy describes the major ethnic differences in craniofacial skull features by categorizing them into four historic groups corresponding with geographic area: (1) Caucasoid (descendants of North American and European individuals), (2) Mongoloid (descendants of peoples from Asia, Polynesia, and Central/South America), (3) Australoid (descendants of pacific islanders, Indonesians, Malaysians, and Australian aborigines), and (4) Negroid (descendants of people from Africa).[17] The defining difference among these categories tends to be variations of the shape of the piriform aperture, the width of the bizygomatic arch, the maxilla, the mandible, the presence of prognathism, and orbital shape.[17] Multiple comprehensive studies on craniofacial differences among ethnic groups have been completed by Leslie Farkas. He analyzed almost 1500 individuals from 18 countries, measuring differences in superficial landmarks and observing variances in bony and soft tissue composition. Describing each of the anatomic differences is beyond the scope of this article; however, it is important to mention that outliers in nearly every measurement were found.[17] This reinforces the idea that even though there are consistent anatomic trends, there is also much variance in facial features within different ethnic groups.

Larrabee and Bevans[17] report several clinical pearls in their article evaluating racial anatomic differences. They note that the most defining characteristics contributing to racial (and individual) appearances are those of the eyes, nasal anatomy, and perioral regions.[17] They describe how Asian eyelids are identified by the lack of supratarsal crease (caused by absent or low skin insertion of the lower levator aponeurosis), epicanthal fold, and narrowed palpebral fissure. Additionally, they note how nasal projection and alar width tend to be inversely related. This relationship is influenced by nasal aperture, cartilage strength and position, and thickness of the skin and soft tissue envelope. Regarding lips, they comment on the increased fullness of Mestizo and African lips than those of Asians and Caucasians.

To our knowledge, there have been no anatomic studies that compare differences in facial muscles or fat compartments among separate racial groups. Because there are notable craniofacial skull differences among ethnic groups, there are changes in the position of the sensory nerves exiting from skeletal foramen. For example, the inferior alveolar nerve exists from the mental foramen, which is located between the first and second premolars in most White and Middle Eastern patients. In comparison, the nerve is located directly below the long axis of the second premolar in Asian races, and inferior to marginally posterior to the second premolar in African races.[18,19]

SKIN THICKNESS

Clinically, an understanding of skin thickness is useful when evaluating dermal atrophy secondary to intralesional corticosteroid injection, for detecting osteoporosis, work-up for acromegaly, and calculations of indirect body fat.[20] Surgically, knowing relative skin thickness at various anatomic sites allows for better reconstructive outcomes when matching donor and recipient tissues. Dermal thickness is vital in surgical planning for reconstruction after cutaneous tumor resection, for needle placement in soft tissue and neurotoxin injections, and other cosmetic procedures. Ultrasound and histometric analyses have most commonly been used to measure in vivo and in vitro skin thickness.

Variability in measurement of absolute skin thickness among individuals makes it difficult to standardize or compare results of different studies. To make a standardized method for clinical analysis of skin thickness, Ha and colleagues[20] created the relative thickness index (RTI). The RTI system works by creating a ratio between the skin thickness of any anatomic site compared with the site of the thinnest portion of skin (eyelid). By examining relative values of skin thickness, using each subject as their own control, the authors were able to calculate consistent ratios of dermal and epidermal thickness from one facial site to another.[20]

A more recent study by Chopra and colleagues[8] expands on the RTI system, where they evaluated skin thickness in 49 predetermined anatomic locations of the face by performing full-thickness punch biopsy samples from 10 human cadaveric heads. Their results showed that the greatest dermal thickness is located at the lower nasal side wall (1969.2 μm) and the thinnest is located at the upper medial eyelid (758.9 μm). The thickest epidermis is the upper lip (62.6 μm), and the thinnest is the posterior auricular skin (29.6 μm). Of note, dermal thickness tended to positively correlate with increased total thickness; however, this pattern was not seen with epidermal thickness.

DIAGNOSTICS

Optical coherence tomography (OCT) is a noninvasive imaging technique that measures reflected infrared light to create a picture, analogous to reflected sound waves used in ultrasound. OCT has been used to measure the thickness of the retina or during cardiac catheterization to produce images of blood vessels. Within dermatology, OCT was first used to diagnose nonmelanoma skin cancers and actinic keratoses in 1997.[21] A hand-held probe emits a low-intensity 1310-nm infrared laser to evaluate tissue of interest. The vertical field of view is a width of up to 10 mm and a depth of 1 to 2 mm with axial resolution of 3 to 15 μm. Single-cell resolution within the skin is not possible, but overall skin architecture is appreciated, including the dermal-epidermal junction, papillary dermis, reticular dermis, blood vessels within the upper dermis, skin appendages, nail unit, and nail plate.

OCT has been clinically useful in the noninvasive diagnosis and presurgical evaluation of tumor margins for nonmelanoma skin cancer.[22,23] Dynamic OCT enables the visualization of cutaneous microvasculature through detection of rapid changes in the interferometric signal of blood flow, useful for the evaluation of vascular lesions.[24] OCT is a compact and portable device that has potential to revolutionize dermatologic surgery and procedures. Real-time imaging may theoretically provide more immediate diagnosis and circumnavigate the need for biopsies and histopathology, thus decreasing potential patient follow-up visits and overall health care expenditure. OCT may assist surgical dissection in anatomic danger zones and improve overall functional outcomes for patients.[25]

CLINICS CARE POINTS

- Blood flow of the skin and subcutaneous tissue of the face is mostly supplied by the external carotid artery with exception to the periorbital region, upper two-thirds of the nose, and central forehead which is supplied by the internal carotid artery.

- Closing a wound perpendicular to RSTL requires twice as much tension when compared with a closure designed parallel to RSTL.

- Layers of the face from superficial to deep include (1) skin, (2) subcutaneous tissue/superficial areolar tissue, (3) superficial fascia/musculoaponeurotic layer, (4) deep areolar tissue/soft tissue spaces, and (5) periosteum/deep fascia.

- The SMAS is a continuous fibromuscular layer that spans the superficial layers of the face and helps transmit, distribute, and amplify facial muscle contractile forces to the skin above.

- Although the etiology is unclear, superficial fat pads have been observed to hypertrophy with age, whereas deep fat compartments are more likely to atrophy.

- Retaining ligaments function to strategically anchor the soft tissue of the face to the deep fascia or skeletal structures beneath and additionally provide conduits for vasculature and branches of the facial nerve.

- Locating soft tissue spaces of the face is surgically important as they provide "safe zones" for dissections as no structures cross within the spaces and the facial nerve branches are protected within the surrounding retaining ligaments.

- The facial nerve is divided into five main branches: (1) frontal (temporal), (2) zygomatic, (3) buccal, (4) marginal mandibular, and (5) cervical. The temporal and mandibular branches pose the greatest risk of injury during cutaneous facial surgery, however understanding the location of each branch will be crucial for navigating surgical approaches.

DISCLOSURE

The authors have nothing to disclose.

REFERENCES

1. Kantor J, Albertini JG, Bordeaux JS, et al. Dermatologic surgery. New York: McGraw Hill/Medical; 2018.

2. Larrabee WF, Makielski KH. Surgical anatomy of the face. New York: Raven Press; 1993.

3. Braz A, Sakuma T, Braz A, et al. Chapter 1, *Facial assessment, dermal fillers facial anatomy and injection techniques*. New York: Thieme Medical Publishers; 2020. https://doi.org/10.1055/B000000255.

4. Larrabee WF, Sutton D. A finite element model of skin deformation. II. An experimental model of skin deformation. Laryngoscope 1986;96(4). https://doi.org/10.1288/00005537-198604000-00013.

5. Cotofana S, Schenck TL, Trevidic P, et al. Midface: clinical anatomy and regional approaches with injectable fillers. Plast Reconstr Surg 2015;136(5). https://doi.org/10.1097/PRS.0000000000001837.

6. Mendelson B, Facelift Wong C-H. Facial anatomy and aging. In: Neligan PC, editor. Plastic surgery, vol. 2, 4th edition. London: Elsevier Inc.; 2018. p. 97–111. Asthetic Surgery.

7. Sykes JM, Riedler KL, Cotofana S, et al. Superficial and deep facial anatomy and its implications for rhytidectomy. Facial Plast Surg Clin North Am 2020; 28(3):243–51.

8. Chopra K, Calva D, Sosin M, et al. A comprehensive examination of topographic thickness of skin in the human face. Aesthetic Surg J 2015;35(8):1007–13.

9. Surek C, Beut J, Stephens R, et al. Pertinent anatomy and analysis for midface volumizing procedures. Plast Reconstr Surg 2015;135(5):818–829e.

10. Wan D, Amirlak B, Rohrich R, et al. The clinical importance of the fat compartments in midfacial aging. Plast Reconstr Surg Glob Open 2013;1(9). https://doi.org/10.1097/GOX.0000000000000035.

11. Gosain AK, Klein MH, Sudhakar PV, et al. A volumetric analysis of soft-tissue changes in the aging midface using high-resolution MRI: implications for facial rejuvenation. Plast Reconstr Surg 2005;115(4):1143–52.

12. Wan D, Amirlak B, Giessler P, et al. The differing adipocyte morphologies of deep versus superficial midfacial fat compartments: a cadaveric study. Plast Reconstr Surg 2014;133(5). https://doi.org/10.1097/PRS.0000000000000100.

13. Trussler AP, Stephan P, Hatef D, et al. The frontal branch of the facial nerve across the zygomatic arch: anatomical relevance of the high-SMAS technique. Plast Reconstr Surg 2010;125(4):1221–30.

14. Moss CJ, Mendelson BC, Taylor GI. Surgical anatomy of the ligamentous attachments in the temple and periorbital regions. Plast Reconstr Surg 2000; 105(4). https://doi.org/10.1097/00006534-200004040-00035.

15. Batra APS, Mahajan A, Gupta K. Marginal mandibular branch of the facial nerve: an anatomical study. Indian J Plast Surg 2010;43(1):60.

16. Chowdhry S, Yoder EM, Cooperman RD, et al. Locating the cervical motor branch of the facial nerve: anatomy and clinical application. Plast Reconstr Surg 2010;126(3):875–9. https://doi.org/10.1097/PRS.0b013e3181e3b374. PMID: 20463628.

17. Larrabee WF, Bevans S. 2 Surgical Anatomy of the Face: Evaluating Racial Differences. In: Cobo R, editor. Ethnic Considerations in Facial Plastic Surgery. 1st edition. New York: Thieme; 2015. 10.1055/b-004-140248.

18. Santini A, Alayan I. A comparative anthropometric study of the position of the mental foramen in three populations. Braz Dent J 2012;212(4). https://doi.org/10.1038/SJ.BDJ.2012.143.

19. Mbajiorgu EF. A study of the position of the mandibular foramen in adult black Zimbabwean mandibles. Cent Afr J Med 2000;46(7):184–90.

20. Ha RY, Nojima K, Adams WP, et al. Analysis of facial skin thickness: defining the relative thickness index. Plast Reconstr Surg 2005;115(6):1769–73.

21. Mehrabi JN, Holmes J, Abrouk M, et al. Vascular characteristics of port wine birthmarks as measured by dynamic optical coherence tomography. J Am Acad Dermatol 2021;85(6):1537–43.

22. Lentsch G, Baugh EG, Lee B, et al. Research techniques made simple: emerging imaging technologies for noninvasive optical biopsy of human skin. J Invest Dermatol 2022;142(5):1243–52.e1.

23. Que SKT. Research techniques made simple: noninvasive imaging technologies for the delineation of basal cell carcinomas. J Invest Dermatol 2016; 136(4):e33–8.

24. Olsen J, Holmes J, Jemec GBE. Advances in optical coherence tomography in dermatology-a review. J Biomed Opt 2018;23(4):1.

25. Fujimoto JG, Pitris C, Boppart SA, et al. Optical coherence tomography: an emerging technology for biomedical imaging and optical biopsy. Neoplasia 2000;2(1–2):9.

Translational Biochemistry of the Skin

Lindsey Voller, MD, Zakia Rahman, MD, FAAD*

KEYWORDS

- Collagen • Elastin • Wound healing • Synthesis • Degradation

KEY POINTS

- Non-invasive aesthetic treatment development and administration mastery begins with an understanding of the translational biochemistry of collagen and elastin in the skin.
- Collagen is the most abundant protein in human skin and undergoes degradation and replacement throughout the course of life.
- Elastin represents a small yet significant component in the skin's ability to maintain biologically healthy stretch and recoil.

INTRODUCTION

The NIH defines translational science as the field of investigation focused on understanding the scientific and operational principles underlying the process of turning observations from the laboratory into clinical diagnostic and therapeutic procedures.[1] An appreciation of the biochemical processes which govern the aesthetic treatments offered to patients in the clinic and the procedure suite is critical to delivering and advancing high-quality patient care. In the specific context of non-invasive skin treatments, most marketable devices, and procedures focus on the upregulation and protection of collagen and elastin, as these two macromolecules play key roles in the skin aging process. A matrix of interwoven dermal collagen fibrils provides structural and mechanical integrity to the epidermis, and combined with elastin, contributes to skin plasticity.[2] Skin that bounces back quickly from mechanical tension, reflects light nicely, and heals quickly from injury subconsciously communicates to others and ourselves that we are healthy internally. Contrary to the outdated ideas that the extracellular matrix is relatively dormant compared to cells, the continual regeneration of this component is essential to healthy tissue. However, with time, the structural support from collagen gradually declines and the elasticity of the skin degenerates. This intrinsic aging can be further advanced by photodamage accumulated over a lifetime, leading to an accelerated appearance of rhytides, pigmentation, and a loss of skin volume. This article discusses the fundamentals of collagen and elastin to provide a basic understanding of the skin and its aging process, as well as the procedures discussed throughout the book herein.

DISCUSSION

Collagen

Collagen, a protein produced exclusively in the animal kingdom, is the predominant component of the dermal extracellular matrix (ECM) and is critical to upholding the structural integrity of human skin, accounting for three-quarters of its dry weight.[3] Collagen is produced by dermal fibroblasts and is first synthesized in the rough endoplasmic reticulum. Each nascent preprocollagen strand consists of a polypeptide α-chain backbone with glycine-X-Y repeats, with X and Y often representing proline and hydroxyproline, respectively. Select proline and lysine residues undergo hydroxylation by prolyl

Department of Dermatology, Stanford University School of Medicine, 450 Broadway Street, Pavilion B, 4th Floor, MC 5338, Redwood City, CA 94603, USA
* Corresponding author. Department of Dermatology, Stanford University School of Medicine, 450 Broadway Street, Pavilion B, 4th Floor, MC 5338, Redwood City, CA 94603, USA
E-mail address: zrahman@stanford.edu

Facial Plast Surg Clin N Am 31 (2023) 443–452
https://doi.org/10.1016/j.fsc.2023.06.009
1064-7406/23/© 2023 Elsevier Inc. All rights reserved.

hydroxylase and lysyl hydroxylase, of which L-ascorbic acid (the most biologically active form of vitamin C) acts as a necessary cofactor.[4] Additional intracellular post-translational modifications occur (eg, glycosylation and formation of disulfide bonds), followed by the coiling of the polypeptide chains into a right-handed triple helix (**Fig. 1**), which may consist of identical (homodimers) or more commonly, dissimilar (heterodimers) chains to form procollagen.[3,5] The triple helix is stabilized by the amino acid pattern Gly-X-Y, electrostatic interactions, and interchain hydrogen bonds.[6] Procollagen undergoes further processing in the Golgi apparatus and is secreted outside of the fibroblast into the extracellular space. Its propeptide N- and C-termini are cleaved by N- and C-proteinases and a tropocollagen molecule is released. Tropocollagen fibrils aggregate, pack in parallel, and covalently cross-link with the assistance of copper-dependent lysyl oxidase to form a mature collagen fiber (**Fig. 2**). The ultimate mechanical properties of collagen are dependent on this final cross-linking process, which works to add resistance under shear stress. The size of these collagen bundles increases in size deeper within the dermis.

There are 28 types of collagen comprising the collagen superfamily, many of which are found in the skin and are highlighted in **Table 1**. Each type of collagen is further subdivided based on its microscopic structure. Importantly, while collagen fibrils are often described by their predominant collagen component (eg, type I collagen fibril), it should be noted that these fibrils often consist of a variety of collagen types, referred to as "heterotopic," and simply named by the subtype which predominates.[6,7] Type I collagen is the dominant protein in human skin, followed by the weaker type III collagen which comprises the predominant component of early granulation tissue. The other fibrillar collagen (type V) and the fibril-associated collagens with interrupted helices (FACITs) (types XII, XIV, XVI, and VI collagens) form trace amounts of the remainders, among the others listed in **Table 1**.[8] Fibrillar collagens play the predominant structural role by contributing to the skin's shape and tensile strength; however, the collagens present in smaller fractions such as FACITs and network collagens are still integral to overall tissue integrity. For instance, although a relative minority as compared to the fibrillar collagen types, type IV collagen is the primary collagen found in the basement membrane and is a well-known cause of Alport syndrome, a rare inherited disorder leading to chronic kidney disease and hearing loss. Type VII collagen is an anchoring fibril critical in the adhesion of the dermal-epidermal junction (DEJ), where it binds types I and III collagen and provides important stability to the interstitial membrane and structures of the basement membrane. Dystrophic epidermolysis bullosa (DEB) and epidermolysis bullosa acquisita (EBA) are two rare blistering disorders involving malfunctions in collagen VII, with DEB related to mutations in the *COL7A1* gene and EBA resulting from autoantibodies formed against collagen VII.[9] Other conditions with well-described collagen mutations include osteogenesis imperfecta (type I collagen), Ehlers-Danlos syndrome (types I and V collagen, primarily), and junctional epidermolysis bullosa (type XVII collagen), among many others which have been described elsewhere extensively.

In addition to its role in the mechanical and structural integrity of the skin, collagen has demonstrated its importance in other cellular functions such as ECM deposition and protein synthesis, which has vital implications in wound healing (Barnes). Immediately following tissue injury, exposed collagen stimulates platelet migration and adherence, contributing to the coagulation cascade and formation of a fibrin clot. The C-terminus of collagen I specifically is involved in the recruitment of endothelial cells.[28] Immune cells and proinflammatory cytokines driven by the wound-healing process such as interleukin (IL)-6, IL-8, and growth factors including transforming growth factor beta (TGF-β) lead to fibroblast migration, stimulating additional collagen deposition (Berman). The simultaneous degradation of collagen by matrix metalloproteinases (MMPs)—a family of zinc-dependent

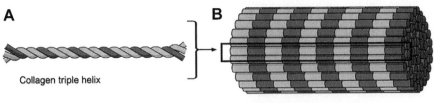

Fig. 1. (*A, B*). Collagen triple helix (*A*) and aggregated, covalently cross-linked collagen fibrils which form a mature collagen fiber (*B*). Illustration created using the Mind the Graph platform at www.mindthegraph.com.

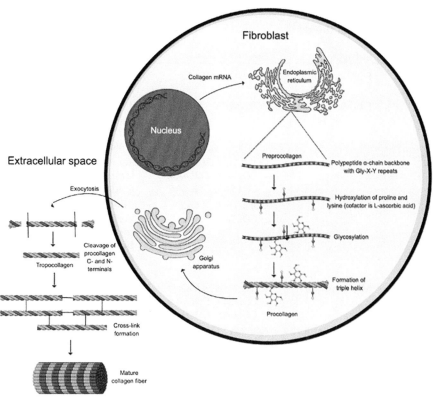

Fig. 2. Simplified schematic of collagen synthesis. Illustration created using the Mind the Graph platform at www. mindthegraph.com.

endopeptidases such as collagenase, gelatinase, stromelysin, and matrilysin—leads to growth factor synthesis which promotes angiogenesis and wound re-epithelialization. The balance of MMPs degrading collagen while a new matrix is deposited leads to the remodeling of the ECM, acquisition of tensile strength, and production of a new structural scaffold. The fibrin clot initially produced at injury onset is replaced by provisional granulation tissue (eg, type III collagen), which is eventually rearranged into type I collagen which results in a stronger scar. Wound remodeling continues for months to up to one year following the initial insult, and the resulting rearrangement is large and abnormal as compared to that of normal dermal collagen. For that reason, the subsequent scar is weaker than uninjured skin, reaching a maximum of 80% of its original strength pre-wound.[8,28]

When the wound healing process occurs aberrantly, hypertrophic or keloid scars may form. Clinically, hypertrophic scars appear as protuberant, firm plaques that are confined to the original scar site and may regress spontaneously. Keloids, in contrast, typically form firm, erythematous, often shiny plaques and/or nodules which grow beyond the boundaries of the initially injured

site, spreading into the normal surrounding skin. As compared to the typical basket-weave collagen found in normal skin, collagen in all types of scars runs perpendicular to the epidermis; however, abnormally thick collagen bundles are seen in keloid scars and may, paradoxically, be thinner in hypertrophic scars.[29] Collagen production is increased in both hypertrophic and keloid scars and exhibit an increased ratio of type I to type III collagen.[30] The increase in collagen and a decrease in elastin accounts for the clinical presentation of a firm plaque. The abnormal collagen remodeling seen in keloid scars, and in a lesser degree in hypertrophic scars, occurs secondarily to the upregulation of proinflammatory factors such as IL-1α, IL-1β, IL-6, and TNF-α in response to tissue trauma, re-wounding (for instance, as with earrings), infection (eg, folliculitis), and/or within regions with high degree of frequent tension, and therefore these scars are thought to represent an inflammatory disorder within the reticular dermis.[31] In contrast to hypertrophic scars, keloid scars can rarely appear spontaneously.[32] Certain patients are at an increased risk of developing hypertrophic or keloid scarring, such as pregnant individuals and adolescents.

Table 1
Types of collagen present in the skin[10]

Collagen Type	Subtype	Gene	Location/Notes
Collagen I[11]	Fibrillar	COL1A1, COL1A2	Most abundant protein in the body, ubiquitous
Collagen III[12]	Fibrillar	COL3A1	Often associated with type I collagen; present in fetal skin, early granulation tissue, vessel walls, lung, liver, spleen
Collagen IV[13]	Network	COL4A1, COL4A2, COL4A3, COL4A4, COL4A5, COL4A6	Basement membranes, including lamina densa of the dermal-epidermal junction (Abreu-Velez)
Collagen V[14]	Fibrillar	COL5A1, COL5A2, COL5A3	Dermis, colon, endometrium, skeletal muscle, lymph node, tonsil, thyroid gland, lung, cornea, bone, fetal membranes, small intestines, testis, cervix, tonsil, parathyroid gland
Collagen VI[15]	Microfibrillar	COL6A1, COL6A2, COL6A3, COL6A4, COL6A5, COL6A6	Dermis, at interface between basement membrane and interstitial matrix
Collagen VII[9]	Anchoring fibril	COL7A1	Binds type I and III collagen, critical for function and stability of ECM[a]
Collagen VIII[16]	Network	COL8A1, COL8A2	Skin, basement membrane of corneal endothelium, bone, brain, cartilage, eye, heart, kidney, liver, lung, muscle, spleen, vascular tissues, ligaments, tendons, nerves
Collagen XII[17]	FACIT[b]	COL12A1	Often associated with type I collagen; component of interstitial matrix
Collagen XIII[18]	Transmembrane	COL13A1	Connective tissue-producing cells, focal adhesions, blood vessels
Collagen XIV[19]	FACIT	COL14A1	Skin, tendon, cornea, articular cartilage, mammary glands
Collagen XVI[20]	FACIT	COL16A1	Skin, cartilage, heart, intestine, arterial walls, kidney, fetal brain, skeletal muscle
Collagen XVII[21]	Transmembrane	COL17A1	Epithelial hemidesmosomes; previously known as bullous pemphigoid antigen (BP180)
Collagen XVIII[22]	Multiplexin	COL18A1	Various basement membrane zones
Collagen XX[23]	FACIT	COL20A1	Embryonic skin, bile ducts, breast, cerebellum, smooth muscle
Collagen XXI[24]	FACIT	COL21A1	Skin, heart, placenta, GI system, kidney, lung, pancreas, lymph nodes
Collagen XXII[25]	FACIT	COL22A1	Skin, myotendinous junctions of heart and skeletal muscle
Collagen XXIII[26]	Transmembrane	COL23A1	Skin, lung, cornea, tendon, amion
Collagen XXVIII[27]	Other	COL28A1	Dermis, calvaria, peripheral nerves, nodes of Ranvier

[a] ECM, extracellular matrix.
[b] FACITs, Fibril-associated collagens with interrupted helices.

Furthermore, patients with darker skin types are 15 times more likely to develop keloids than those with lighter skin types, which may suggest a genetic predisposition to abnormal scarring.[31] In addition to undesirable cosmesis, keloids may lead to discomfort such as pain, pruritus, or burning. If large enough, keloids can also restrict range of motion. Therefore, treatment and more importantly the prevention of these scars, is of utmost importance to patient care. Management of hypertrophic and keloid scarring is multifactorial and discussed elsewhere (see Jill S. Waibel and Emily Sedaghat's article, "Scar Therapy of Skin," in this issue).

Elastin

While collagen provides the skin with its tensile strength, elastin is responsible for the critical ability of the skin—in addition to vital structures such as the lungs, aorta, arterial blood vessels, ligaments, and tendons—to glide, stretch, and recoil after being deformed by external force. Elastic fibers account for significantly less dermal dry weight as compared to collagen (only 2–4%), but play a significant role in skin elasticity and resilience.[33,34] They consist predominantly of an inner dense core of elastin with an outer layer of fibrillin-rich microfibrils.[35] Elastin is produced by fibroblasts in a process termed elastogenesis. Following the transcription of ELN, mature, soluble tropoelastin mRNA is translated into the protein tropoelastin in the rough endoplasmic reticulum. Tropoelastin consists of alternating hydrophobic and hydrophilic domains; the hydrophobic domains are rich in non-polar amino acids, while the hydrophilic domains contain a predominant component of alanine and lysine-rich cross-links.[36] Tropelastin interacts with elastin-binding protein (EBP), which protects tropoelastin from degradation, and the tropoelastin-EBP complex is secreted from the fibroblast. In the extracellular environment, tropoelastin polypeptides bind to the fibroblast cell surface and aggregate into globules/spherules in a microassembly phase called coacervation.[34] Tropoelastin multimers form extensive covalent cross-links (desmosines) under the oxidative influence of copper-dependent lysyl oxidase, the same enzyme involved in collagen cross-linking discussed previously. Cross-linked tropoelastin remains on the fibroblast surface until additional tropoelastin polypeptides associate with microfibrils, which consist of proteins such as fibrillins 1 and 2, fibulins 1, 2, 3, 4, and 5, and others.[33] The association of tropoelastin with microfibrils results in the final alignment and scaffolding of elastic fibers (**Fig. 3**).[10] The fibers are arranged in varying directions and their orientation differs throughout the dermis. Within the more superficial papillary dermis, specific elastic fibers termed oxytalan fibers are oriented perpendicular to the DEJ, which connect to a finer network of elaunin fibers in the lower papillary dermis. Deeper within the reticular dermis, elastin fibers are the primary component and run parallel to the DEJ. The resulting product is an intricate network of interwoven elastic fibers within the dermis which can undergo multiple cycles of stretch and recoil while minimally changing its overall structure (**Fig. 4**).[34,37] The epidermis, in contrast, is largely devoid of elastic fibers, although cultured keratinocytes have been shown to express low levels of elastin gene at low levels.[33]

Collagen, Elastin, and the Aging Skin

Collagen levels gradually decrease with time and their loss is accelerated by photodamage. Oxidative stress accumulated over a lifetime leads to abnormal synthesis and increased degradation of collagen. As compared to younger skin, collagen in intrinsically aged skin is coarse, fragmented, and disorganized, and has a higher proportion of collagen III.[28] Regarding photoaging specifically, UV radiation upregulates mitogen-activated protein kinases (MAPKs) in the epidermis and upper dermis, which phosphorylate the transcription factor, c-Jun. c-Jun enters the nucleus, partners with c-Fos, and induces transcription factor AP-1, which interferes with collagenesis and impairs the effects of TGF-β.[38] MMPs are also upregulated following exposure to UV radiation. MMP-1 is induced by UV light and cleaves fibrillar collagen types I and III.[39] As degraded fibrils accumulate, fibroblasts sense the low mechanical stress in the extracellular environment and respond by reducing collagen production and increasing levels of MMPS, which cleave the collagenous ECM. The upregulation of MMP expression coupled with a downregulation of collagen production leads to an ongoing cycle of oxidative stress, fragmentation of collagen fibrils, and ultimately decreased collagenesis.[38] This MMP-mediated damage is cumulative and potentiates with subsequent exposures to sunlight. This process of photoaging mediated by chronic exposure to UV light accounts for approximately 80% of the effects of facial aging.[40] Additional areas which are chronically exposed to sunlight such as the dorsal hands, forearms, and neck are also particularly susceptible to premature aging.

Elastin undergoes similar changes in response to intrinsic- and photoaging. Elastolytic enzymes called elastases cause degradation of microfibrils and shortening of elastic fibers, resulting in an

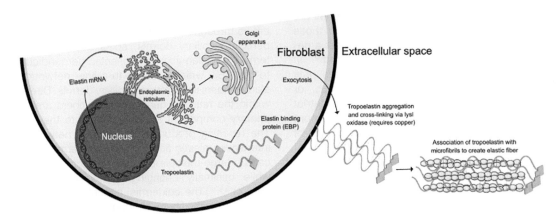

Fig. 3. Simplified schematic of elastin synthesis. Illustration created using the Mind the Graph platform at www.mindthegraph.com.

overall disruption to the elastic fiber network; fibulin-5 may also be lost.[34,41] However, unlike collagen which is continuously regenerated, the gene expression and resulting protein synthesis of elastin occurs only within a narrow window from late embryonic development through adolescence; in fact, their half-life is around 70 years, relatively comparable to the human lifespan.[36] In other words, new elastin is not produced in adult life. Elastic fibers are therefore significantly more difficult to regenerate, and treatments are therefore often focused on their preservation rather than restoration.

Clinically, intrinsically aged skin appears thin, finely wrinkled, with exaggerated lines of expression, although with a generally clear complexion and uniform pigmentation (**Fig. 5**). Redundant, loose, or sagging skin from loss of elastic fibers

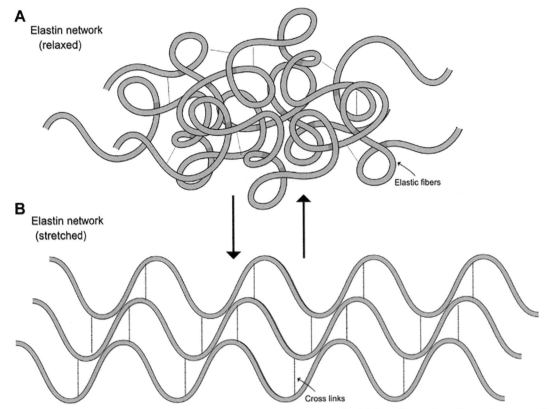

Fig. 4. (*A, B*). Schematic of elastin network in a relaxed (*A*) and stretched (*B*) configuration. Illustration created using the Mind the Graph platform at www.mindthegraph.com.

can also be seen. Photodamaged skin with solar elastosis, in contrast, typically has a thickened and leathery appearance, with dyspigmentation and the accumulation of benign skin neoplasms such as solar lentigines (**Fig. 6**). Additional clinical signs of ECM degradation include the appearance of actinic purpura, atrophic acne scars, skin crepiness (most evident on the lateral cheeks and neck), striae (a form of atrophic scarring), cellulite, and horizontal neck rhytides. Histopathologically, photodamage manifests as an accumulation of amorphous elastin material termed solar elastosis, or the accumulation of large, disorganized elastic fibers replacing normal papillary dermis (**Fig. 7**). Elastosis secondary to cigarette smoking has also been well-described and similarly leads to the degradation of elastic fibers within the dermis, resulting in deep wrinkles particularly around the mouth and periorbital region.[40] Given that external factors such as photodamage and cigarette smoking hasten the appearance of fine lines and wrinkles, it is critical to educate patients on the modifiable factors which can result in accelerating biological aging.

Roles of Collagen and Elastin in Non-invasive Skin Treatments

As the majority of non-invasive skin treatments focus on an aspect of the wound healing process, a comprehensive understanding of the structure and synthesis of collagen and elastin is critical to performing procedures targeting their upregulation and protection. Topical vitamin A in the form of retinoids, for instance, inhibit MMP expression and therefore stimulate collagen synthesis. This effect is mediated by retinoic acid and retinoid X receptors (RAR and RXR, respectively), which are nuclear hormone receptors that bind synthetic retinoids selectively.[42] Homo- or heterodimers of RAR and RXR, along with their specific retinoid, translocate

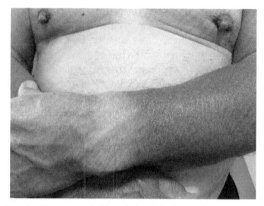

Fig. 6. Photoaged skin of the left dorsal forearm and hand with the accumulation of solar lentigines, solar purpura, and atrophy; note the contrast to the intrinsically aged skin of the chest and abdomen. The left dorsal wrist skin where the wristband of this individual's watch normally resides, demonstrates a midway point of progressive aging dependent on the degree of sun exposure.

to the nucleus, bind to promoters, and modulate gene transcription of retinoid-sensitive genes. Additional examples of the downstream effects of retinoids include the inhibition of AP-1 and c-Jun and alteration of TGF-β expression ultimately leading to an increase in collagen synthesis. Topical retinoids have also been shown to result in fibrillin restoration in the skin which acts a scaffold for elastin. Increased vascularity and angiogenesis from retinoid treatment may additionally contribute to a decrease in the appearance of rhytides.[42]

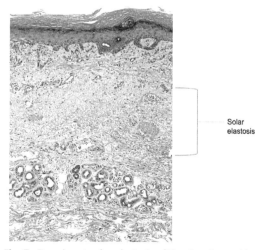

Solar elastosis

Fig. 7. Prominent solar elastosis of the dermis resulting from chronic photodamage. Adapted from Wikimedia Commons (Solar elastosis - intermed mag, by Nephron. Retrieved from: https://commons.wikimedia.org/wiki/File:Solar_elastosis_-_intermed_mag.jpg.)

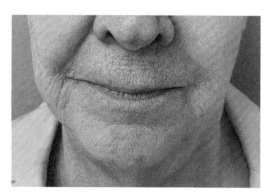

Fig. 5. Intrinsically aged and solar elastosis in skin of the lower face, exhibiting yellow appearance, wrinkling, and exaggeration of expression lines.

Another important topical in the upregulation of collagenesis is L-ascorbic acid, the most biologically active form of vitamin C, which functions as an antioxidant that neutralizes free radicals in the environment and after exposure to UV radiation.[43] As discussed previously, vitamin C is a necessary cofactor in the hydroxylation of proline and lysine in collagen synthesis and stabilization; similar to retinoids. Vitamin C also activates transcription factors involved in neocollagenesis, stabilizes pro-collagen messenger RNA (mRNA), and inhibits AP-1 activation, all of which lead to an overall increase in collagen gene expression.[44]

Outside of topical therapies, noninvasive skin procedures are effective treatments which work similarly to promote neocollagenesis. Injectables fillers such as hyaluronic acid, calcium hydroxyapatite, and poly-l-lactic acid have been shown to upregulate fibroblast activity around the injected filler and increase collagen and elastin deposition.[45–47] Microneedling harnesses a pulsating circular array of needles to create controlled micro-injuries within the skin, stimulating the release of dermal growth factors, fibroblast activation, and subsequent collagen deposition while preserving the structural integrity of the epidermis.[48] Broadband light, also known as intense pulse light, has also led to improvements in skin rejuvenation and may lead to more organized, uniform distribution of collagen fibers.[49] Photothermal laser tissue interaction with fractional or full field ablative (CO2 10,600 nm, Er:YAG 2,940 nm) and non-ablative lasers (Diode 1440/1470 nm, Thulium 1927 nm, Er:Glass 1550 nm) have demonstrated the upregulation of wound healing resulting in the elimination of damaged epidermis and dermis as well as the upregulation of collagen and elastin production.[50,51] These procedures will be discussed in further detail extensively throughout the book herein.

Future Directions

The upregulation of collagen and preservation of elastin are clearly critical to achieving skin rejuvenation. Looking to the future, new developments in the realm of multi-omics may represent an interesting pathway to expand upon currently established therapies. Through analysis of the genome, transcriptome, and epigenome, recent work by Gill and colleagues[52] has demonstrated the upregulation of collagen production following the application of maturation phase transient reprogramming to dermal fibroblasts. The expression of genes for collagen I and IV were restored to youthful levels following transient reprogramming, demonstrating that fibroblasts can potentially be rejuvenated transcriptionally and at the protein level in regards to collagen production. This relatively nascent field is ripe for future research, and a fundamental understanding of these multi-omics processes is necessary to optimize current treatments and guide directions for the development of future technology in the aesthetic space.

Additional interesting recent research has involved a topical gene delivery system for collagen replacement; beremagene geperpavec (B-VEC), an investigational herpes simplex virus type 1 (HSV-1)–based, topical gene therapy, designed to restore functional C7 protein through delivery of COL7A1 was approved in 2023 for the treatment of dystrophic epidermolysis bullosa.[53] This paves the way for potential future applications of gene therapy to address aesthetic loss of collagen and elastin in the skin.

SUMMARY

Collagen and elastin clearly play critical roles in maintaining and restoring a youthful skin appearance. This article summarized the biochemical processes involving the synthesis, upregulation, and maintenance of these important macromolecules to provide an understanding of the basics of non-invasive skin treatments. A multitude of therapies exist which build on the principles discussed throughout this article, which will aid clinicians in delivering and enhancing patient care.

CLINICS CARE POINTS

- Collagen and elastin are synthesized by dermal fibroblasts and play integral roles in maintaining structural integrity and resilience of the skin.

- Both collagen and elastin degenerate with intrinsic aging, and their degradation is -accelerated by photodamage accumulated following exposure to ultraviolet radiation.

- The majority of noninvasive skin modalities is focused on the upregulation and/or preservation of collagen and elastin.

- Future therapies including multi-omics and topical gene delivery systems for collagen replacement are being investigated and pave the way for future directions in the field of aesthetics.

DISCLOSURE

Dr L. Voller: None. Dr Z. Rahman: Consultant and Advisory Board Allergan Aesthetics.

REFERENCES

1. National Institutes of Health. Transforming Translational Science. Available at: https://ncats.nih.gov/files/translation-factsheet.pdf. (2019, accessed 8 June 2023).

2. Zhang Z, Zhu H, Zheng Y, et al. The effects and mechanism of collagen peptide and elastin peptide on skin aging induced by D-galactose combined with ultraviolet radiation. J Photochem Photobiol B Biol 2020;210:111964.

3. Shoulders MD, Raines RT. Collagen structure and stability. Annu Rev Biochem 2009;78:929–58.

4. Telang P. Vitamin C in dermatology. Indian Dermatol Online J 2013;4:143.

5. Karsdal MA. Biochemistry of Collagens, Laminins and Elastin. p. xxiii–xliv.

6. Ricard-Blum S. The collagen family. Cold Spring Harb Perspect Biol 2011;3:1–19.

7. Bruckner P. Suprastructures of extracellular matrices: Paradigms of functions controlled by aggregates rather than molecules. Cell Tissue Res 2010;339:7–18.

8. Barnes M. Update on Collagens: What You Need to Know and Consider. Plast Surg Nurs 2019;39:112–5.

9. Mortensen JH, Karsdal MA. Type VII collagen. 2nd edition. Elsevier Inc; 2019. https://doi.org/10.1016/B978-0-12-817068-7.00007-0.

10. Nyström A, Bruckner-Tuderman L. Biology of the extracellular matrix. In: Bolognia JL, Schaffer JV, Cerroni L, editors. Dermatology. Fourth Edition. Elsevier; 2018. p. 1675–89.

11. Henriksen K, Karsdal MA. Type I collagen. Second Edition. Elsevier Inc; 2019. https://doi.org/10.1016/B978-0-12-817068-7.00001-X.

12. Nielsen MJ, Villesen IF, Sinkeviciute D, et al. Type III collagen. Second Edition. Elsevier Inc; 2019. https://doi.org/10.1016/B978-0-12-817068-7.00003-3.

13. Sand JMB, Genovese F, Gudmann NS, et al. Type IV collagen. Second Edition. Elsevier Inc; 2019. https://doi.org/10.1016/B978-0-12-817068-7.00004-5.

14. Leeming DJ, Karsdal MA. Type V collagen. Second Edition. Elsevier Inc; 2019. https://doi.org/10.1016/B978-0-12-817068-7.00005-7.

15. Sun S, Genovese F, Karsdal MA. Type VI collagen. Second Edition. Elsevier Inc; 2019. https://doi.org/10.1016/B978-0-12-817068-7.00006-9. t.

16. Hansen NUB, Gudmann NS, Karsdal MA. Type VIII collagen. Second Edition. Elsevier Inc; 2019. https://doi.org/10.1016/B978-0-12-817068-7.00008-2.

17. Mortensen JH, Manon-Jensen T, Karsdal MA. Type XII collagen. Second Edition. Elsevier Inc; 2019. https://doi.org/10.1016/B978-0-12-817068-7.00012-4.

18. Siebuhr AS, Thudium CS, Karsdal MA. Type XIII collagen. Second Edition. Elsevier Inc; 2019. https://doi.org/10.1016/B978-0-12-817068-7.00013-6.

19. Lindholm M, Manon-Jensen T, Karsdal MA. Type XIV collagen. Second Edition. Elsevier Inc; 2019. https://doi.org/10.1016/B978-0-12-817068-7.00014-8.

20. Sand JMB, Jensen C, Karsdal MA. Type XVI collagen. Second Edition. Elsevier Inc; 2019. https://doi.org/10.1016/B978-0-12-817068-7.00016-1.

21. Sun S, Karsdal MA. Type XVII collagen. Second Edition. Elsevier Inc; 2019. https://doi.org/10.1016/B978-0-12-817068-7.00017-3.

22. Pehrsson M, Bager CL, Karsdal MA. Type XVIII collagen. Second Edition. Elsevier Inc; 2019. https://doi.org/10.1016/B978-0-12-817068-7.00018-5.

23. Willumsen N, Nissen NI, Karsdal MA. Type XX collagen. Second Edition. Elsevier Inc; 2019. https://doi.org/10.1016/B978-0-12-817068-7.00020-3.

24. Kehlet SN, Jessen H, Karsdal MA. Type XXI collagen. Second Edition. Elsevier Inc; 2019. https://doi.org/10.1016/B978-0-12-817068-7.00021-5.

25. Kehlet SN, Jessen H, Karsdal MA. Type XXII collagen. Second Edition. Elsevier Inc; 2019. https://doi.org/10.1016/B978-0-12-817068-7.00022-7.

26. Kehlet SN, Jessen H, Karsdal MA. Type XXIII collagen. Second Edition. Elsevier Inc; 2019. https://doi.org/10.1016/B978-0-12-817068-7.00023-9.

27. Sparding N, Arvanitidis A, Karsdal MA. Type XXVIII collagen. Second Edition. Elsevier Inc; 2019. https://doi.org/10.1016/B978-0-12-817068-7.00028-8.

28. Mathew-Steiner SS, Roy S, Sen CK. Collagen in wound healing. Bioengineering 2021;8(5):63.

29. Verhaegen PDHM, Van Zuijlen PPM, Pennings NM, et al. Differences in collagen architecture between keloid, hypertrophic scar, normotrophic scar, and normal skin: an objective histopathological analysis. Wound Repair Regen 2009;17:649–56.

30. Berman B, Maderal A, Raphael B. Keloids and hypertrophic scars: pathophysiology, classification, and treatment. Dermatologic Surg 2017;43:S3–18.

31. Ogawa R. Keloid and hypertrophic scars are the result of chronic inflammation in the reticular dermis. Int J Mol Sci 2017;18(3):606. Epub ahead of print 2017.

32. Jfri A, Rajeh N, Karkashan E. A case of multiple spontaneous keloid scars. Case Rep Dermatol 2015;7:156–60.

33. Uitto J, Li Q, Urban Z. The complexity of elastic fibre biogenesis in the skin–a perspective to the clinical heterogeneity of cutis laxa. Exp Dermatol 2013;22:88–92.

34. Baumann L, Bernstein EF, Weiss AS, et al. Clinical relevance of elastin in the structure and function of skin. Aesthetic Surg journal Open forum 2021;3:ojab019.

35. Schräder CU, Heinz A, Majovsky P, et al. Elastin is heterogeneously cross-linked. J Biol Chem 2018;293:15107–19.

36. Wang K, Meng X, Guo Z. Elastin structure, synthesis, regulatory mechanism and relationship with cardiovascular diseases. Front Cell Dev Biol 2021;9:1–10.

37. Ozsvar J, Yang C, Cain SA, et al. Tropoelastin and elastin assembly. Front Bioeng Biotechnol 2021;9: 1–11.

38. Rittié L, Fisher GJ. Natural and sun-induced aging of human skin. Cold Spring Harb Perspect Med 2015; 5:1–14.

39. Fisher GJ, Kang S, Varani J, et al. Mechanisms of photoaging and chronological skin aging. Arch Dermatol 2002;138:1462–70.

40. Langton AK, Sherratt MJ, Griffiths CEM, et al. A new wrinkle on old skin: the role of elastic fibres in skin ageing. Int J Cosmet Sci 2010;32:330–9.

41. Shin JW, Kwon SH, Choi JY, et al. Molecular mechanisms of dermal aging and antiaging approaches. Int J Mol Sci 2019;20(9):2126.

42. Darlenski R, Surber C, Fluhr JW. Topical retinoids in the management of photodamaged skin: From theory to evidence-based practical approach. Br J Dermatol 2010;163:1157–65.

43. Enescu CD, Bedford LM, Potts G, et al. A review of topical vitamin C derivatives and their efficacy. J Cosmet Dermatol 2022;21:2349–59.

44. Al-Niaimi F, Chiang NYZ. Topical vitamin C and the skin: mechanisms of action and clinical applications. J Clin Aesthet Dermatol 2017;10:14–7.

45. Wu GT, Kam J, Bloom JD. Hyaluronic acid basics and rheology. Facial Plast Surg Clin North Am 2022;30:301–8.

46. Paliwal S, Fagien S, Sun X, et al. Skin extracellular matrix stimulation following injection of a hyaluronic acid-based dermal filler in a rat model. Plast Reconstr Surg 2014 Dec;134(6):1224–33.

47. Coleman KM, Voigts R, DeVore DP, et al. Neocollagenesis after injection of calcium hydroxylapatite composition in a canine model. Dermatol Surg 2008;34(Suppl 1):S53–5.

48. Wamsley CE, Kislevitz M, Barillas J, et al. A single-center trial to evaluate the efficacy and tolerability of four microneedling treatments on fine lines and wrinkles of facial and neck skin in subjects with fitzpatrick skin types I-IV: an objective assessment using noninvasive devices and 0.33-mm. Aesthetic Surg J 2021;41:NP1603–18.

49. Chang ALS, Bitter PH, Qu K, et al. Rejuvenation of gene expression pattern of aged human skin by broadband light treatment: a pilot study. J Invest Dermatol 2013;133:394–402.

50. Kuo T, Speyer MT, Ries WR, et al. Collagen thermal damage and collagen synthesis after cutaneous laser resurfacing. Lasers Surg Med 1998;23(2): 66–71.

51. Laubach HJ, Tannous Z, Anderson RR, et al. Skin responses to fractional photothermolysis. Lasers Surg Med 2006;38(2):142–9.

52. Gill D, Parry A, Santos F, et al. Multi-omic rejuvenation of human cells by maturation phase transient reprogramming. Elife 2022;11:1–23.

53. Guide SV, Gonzalez ME, Bağcı IS, et al. Trial of Beremagene Geperpavec (B-VEC) for Dystrophic Epidermolysis Bullosa. N Engl J Med 2022;387:2211–9.

Scar Therapy of Skin

Jill S. Waibel, MD[a],*, Hannah Waibel, BS[a,b,c,d], Emily Sedaghat, MD[e]

KEYWORDS

- Scars • Scar therapy • Acne scars • Surgical scars • Burn and trauma scars
- Early intervention scars • Laser-assisted drug delivery scars

KEY POINTS

- Contemporary scar therapy has evolved rapidly with multiple treatment modalities including topical, intralesional, surgical, and energy-based therapies developed to restore damage to more normal skin.
- Early intervention in wounds can mitigate and even prevent scar formation.
- Current technologies permit successful treatment of various types of scars.

 Video content accompanies this article at http://www.facialplastic.theclinics.com.

INTRODUCTION: SCARS AND SCAR THERAPIES

Scars are the result of wounds that affect millions of people in the world and are prevalent in both civilians and wounded warriors injured in military combat. Scar treatment is important in medicine and belongs to all medical professionals (Videos 1 and 2). The goal of treating scars includes maximizing the functional independence of patients, improving the patient's quality of life, and enabling patients to get back as close as possible to their preinjury state. The initial injury may be caused by trauma, surgery, burns, or inflammatory skin disease (acne, lupus, and so on). Treatment of acute wounds includes systemic stabilization and surgical intervention. Despite excellent trauma and surgical care, patients continue to have functional impairments and difficult symptoms from scars. Severe cutaneous scars are disfiguring and have many associated symptomatology including pruritus, pain, decreased function, and restricted range of motion. The new goal for scar treatment is that definitive reconstruction ends with recovery of optimal appearance and function.

Multiple therapeutic options have been used to improve scars.[1] Contemporary scar therapy has evolved rapidly with a focus on tissue rehabilitation. There are multiple treatment modalities including topical, intralesional, surgical, and energy-based therapies developed to restore damaged to more normal skin. Multiple scar treatment options are listed in **Table 1** (**Fig. 1**).

Treatment of scars necessitates a multiprocedural and multispecialty approach by a team of scar-experienced medical professionals. There are many ideas and innovations showing great promise in scar therapy, but laser-based therapy has undoubtedly been the most rapid and impactful advance in scar treatment in modern days. Lasers have given scar patients the option for further scar improvements in function, symptoms, and cosmesis. Lasers are a scientifically precise and effective treatment modality to rehabilitate and improve scars.[2] In recent consensus guidelines lasers are considered first-line therapy in the management of scars.[3] Laser has added a powerful tool to improve scar deformities and symptoms.[4]

Funding source: none.
a Southern Methodist University; b Private Practice: Miami Dermatology and Laser Institute, 7800 Southwest 87th Avenue Suite B200, Miami, FL 33173, USA; c Baptist Hospital, Miami, FL, USA; d Dermatology Faculty, Miller School of Medicine, University of Miami; e 118800 Bird Road, Suite 416, Miami, FL 33175, USA
* Corresponding author.
E-mail address: jwaibelmd@miamidermlaser.com

Table 1
Scar treatment options

Current Scar Therapies	Adjunctive Scar Therapies
Topical silicone materials—gels, gel sheeting, sprays	Physical therapy
Novel wound dressings and supports	Psychological and psychiatric therapy
Topical balms—vitamin E, corticosteroids, paper tape	Emerging regenerative medicine—not FDA approved yet
Intralesional injections—triamcinolone acetonide, 5-fluoruracil, bleomycin, retinoic acid, botulinum toxin A	
Surgical revision	
Laser therapy	
Laser-assisted drug delivery	
Autologous fat grafting	
Hyperbaric oxygen therapy	

Scarring is a tissue response, acquired during the second trimester of fetal development at the same time of cellular immunity.[5] Scar tissue has increased vascular and lymphatic channels as well as changes in collagen structure compared with normal skin. However, in scars the blood vessels, lymphatics, and collagen often are in a chaotic array with resultant decreased physiologic function.

It took a Nobel prize winner, Albert Einstein, to form the concept of stimulated emission of radiation in 1917. Einstein postulated the creation of a stream of uniform photons could create a laser beam. The first carbon dioxide (CO_2) laser was invented by Patel of Bell Labs in 1964.[6]

We continue to gain understanding of the biological basis by which scars improve after laser therapy. The scar improvements occur in the epidermis, dermis, and in the adnexal skin structures. Many patients report immediate improvement in pruritus, pain, and increased range of motion within hours to weeks after even one treatment session. After laser therapy typically the skin heals first with improvement of dyschromias followed in time with improvements in texture and topography.

SURGERY AND LASER SYNERGY FOR TREATMENT OF SCARS

The treatment of scars is a multispecialty endeavor. A combination approach with medical experts yields optimal scar improvements. If an injury heals in the presence of tension, hypertrophy often ensues. Understanding the role of tension in the development of a scar is essential to design a successful treatment strategy. If there is significant hypertrophy or contracture present in a scar, surgical intervention is necessary to relieve the tension or there is a high likelihood the scar with reform. Z-plasties remain an important partner with laser in the treatment of contracture scars (**Fig. 2**). After tension relief, hypertrophic and contracture scars are more elastic with new remodeling of collagen and are more amenable to treatment with laser. However, if a scar has had initial fractional laser therapy this often makes surgical intervention easier to perform due to thinner and more pliable collagen bundles.

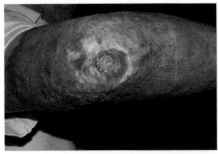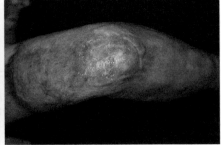

Fig. 1. Before and after 4 combination laser treatments of pulsed dye laser, 1927 nm thulium laser fractional ablative laser followed by 2 months of hyperbaric oxygen to heal ulcer on elbow.

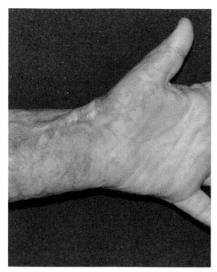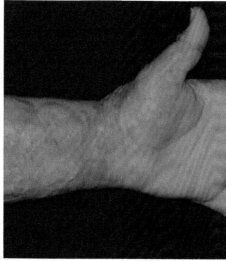

Fig. 2. Before and after a series of punch biopsies and 3 fractional ablative CO2 laser treatments on acne scars.

APPROACH TO TREATMENT OF CUTANEOUS SCARS

In the initial evaluation of the scar the physician should determine what characteristics the scar possesses and then choose therapies to address these issues. Some factors to consider when treating scars include the thickness of the scar, age of scar, body location of the scar and tension forces, skin type of the patient, and comorbid medical conditions. Next determine if a scar is hypertrophic, keloid, contracture, atrophic, or a combination. Then dyschromia of a scar should be evaluated for erythema, hyperpigmentation, and hypopigmentation. Often severe scars have multiple of these characteristics within the same scar. Our approach is to first use nonablative laser to treat vascular and pigmented components of the scar and then to use fractional ablative devices for ablation of scar tissue, coagulation of microvasculature, and stimulation of subsequent neocollagenesis, followed by a beneficial laser-assisted delivery drug. The fractional ablative devices are the mainstay of therapy due to their ability to improve all scar types. Repeated laser sessions can occur until the patient and/or physician is satisfied. After, healing silicone gel sheeting or compression therapy is reinitiated and used until scar reaches optimal improvement.

CLINICAL INDICATIONS AND TREATMENT RECOMMENDATIONS

Treating cutaneous scars requires proper diagnosis of scars as well as an understanding of their histology and biology. Most scars result from acne, surgery, trauma, or burns. Techniques and settings for each of these scars is reviewed in this chapter based on cause of scar.

Acne Scars

Acne vulgaris is the most common inflammatory dermatosis in the world. Although it presents in 95% to 100% of men and 83% to 85% of women during puberty,[7] acne commonly extends into adulthood.[8] Acne can result in scarring, postinflammatory erythema (PIE), and postinflammatory hyperpigmentation (PIH). Postinflammatory dyschromia poses a significant psychological burden on acne patients, often accounting for greater concern than the original acne lesions. For this reason, the management and treatment of postinflammatory dyschromia represents a substantial proportion of the clinical, emotional, and economic burden associated with acne vulgaris.[9] Importantly, this burden most commonly and disproportionately affects skin-of-color patients[10] and can be the most distressing aspect of acne in skin-of-color patients with Fitzpatrick skin phototypes III to VI. Laser therapy with nonablative lasers can help significantly with PIE and PIH (**Fig. 3**). Acneiform scars are the result of compromised collagen production during the natural wound healing process, resulting in cutaneous depressions. Topographic features of acne scarring include perpendicular bundles of collagen that anchor the skin of the scars down. Most of the patients have facial atrophic scars including boxcar, ice pick, and rolling types. These scars result from loss of collagen from inflammation during the wound healing process of acneiform lesions.

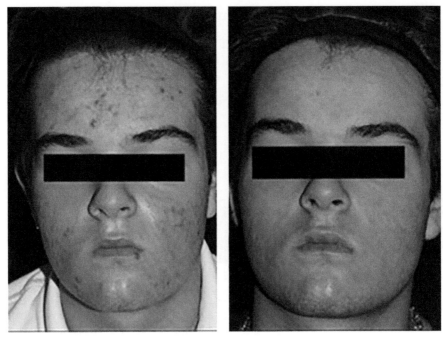

Fig. 3. Before and after 2 treatments of pulsed dye laser and nonablative 1550 nm fractional laser for postinflammatory erythema, resulting in improvement of color and texture of skin.

The goal of laser resurfacing is to create neocollagenesis in the areas of collagen loss (**Fig. 4**). Given the dermal pathology present with acne scarring, particularly with atrophic scars, treatment modalities should optimally be capable of affecting dermal remodeling at least 1 mm below the skin. Patients with acne scars on their chest and back are often hypertrophic or keloidal.

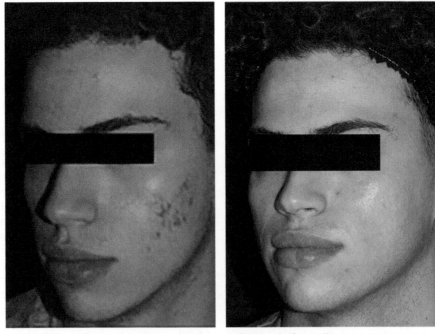

Fig. 4. Combined PDL and fractional ablative CO_2 laser. Before and after rolling acne scars status postablative fractional laser treatment with subcision and laser-assisted delivery of poly-L-lactic acid.

Treatment options for acne scars include those listed in **Box 1**.

Treatment of acne scars has traditionally been challenging; however, with the advent of deep-reaching fractional lasers greater success has been achieved. Superficial approaches include glycolic acid chemical peels and topical tretinoin and topical hydroquinone for skin surface improvement and pigmentary variation. Moderate approaches to address deeper scars include punch biopsy and closure, z-plasty transposition flap, fat polysaccharide matrix or collagen, scar subcision, dermabrasion, CO_2 laser resurfacing, and most recently, fractional photothermolysis.[11] An international consensus recommendation for the energy-based devices for the treatment of acne scars was published in 2022 with multiple algorithms and recommendations.[7] In these recommendations, ablative fractional lasers played a prominent role. Ablative fractional CO_2 laser has been well studied for acne scarring. In a case series of 2 to 3 treatment sessions for moderate-to-severe acne scarring, clinical improvements of 26% to 50% were achieved in texture, atrophy, and overall improvements and on topographic analysis. Improvements in scar depths of 43% to 79.9% were achieved, with a mean depth improvement of 66.8%. Greater degree of improvement seen with ablative fractional laser technology as opposed to previous studies with nonablative fractional laser technology resulted from deeper dermal penetration of the fractionated CO_2 and Erbium:YAG devices. Particularly, they noted that patients treated for deeper scars on the cheeks with higher energy levels on the second and third treatments received the highest improvement scores.[12] Side effects with the ablative fractional device were mild to moderate, including posttreatment erythema, edema, and petechiae,

---

Box 1
Acne scar treatments

Punch biopsies—rolling and boxcar

Z-plasty

Microcoring

Subcision

Fractional laser resurfacing

Microneedling radiofrequency

Fillers and biostimulators

Injectable antimetabolites

Retinoids

Dermabrasion

---

all of which resolved within 7 days after each treatment. Correlating with these clinical data, in vivo studies by Hantash and colleagues with this device have shown tissue ablation and thermal effects as deep as 1 mm into this skin, likely accounting for the effect on moderate-to-severe acne scarring observed.[13]

Another study with the fractionated CO_2 laser for the treatment of acne scarring 15 subjects underwent up to 3 treatments. Patients with a diversity of skin types (I–V) were treated with no complications of short- or long-term hyperpigmentation reported. Eighty-seven percent of subjects sustained significant improvement in the appearance of acne scarring at 3-month follow-up visits. All subjects reported transient erythema, which resolved in the first 2 weeks after treatment.[14] Ablative fractional devices work for all skin types. In a prospective study in 5 Asian patients of skin phototype IV, with moderate to severe atrophic acne scarring, 2 sessions of an ablative fractional CO_2 laser treatment were performed 6 to 8 weeks apart.[15]

Surgical Scars

All surgical scars improve with fractional ablative laser. First one must evaluate if the surgical scar is elevated (hypertrophic) or depressed (atrophic). The thicker hypertrophic scars need deeper treatment depths, whereas more atrophic scars can be treated more superficially. Early surgical scars with significant erythema respond to vascular lasers with or without same day treatment of fractional lasers (**Fig. 5**). In a study of 23 Korean women with thyroidectomy scars single session of 2 passes with a fractional CO_2 laser with a pulse energy of 50 mJ and density of 100 spots/cm^2 was performed. Treatments were performed 2 to 3 weeks after surgery.[16]

Burn and Traumatic Scars

Burn and traumatic scars are typically first treated by the burn and reconstructive surgeons to stabilize the injuries. The surgical tools are listed in **Box 2**. After surgical intervention laser therapy should be used. Erythematous, hypertrophic scars are seen frequently in the first year after injury. Vascular-specific lasers and light devices, especially the 595-nm pulsed dye laser (PDL), are already well established for such applications, and its use has been highlighted in 2 recent reviews.[17,18] PDL may be applied alone for small hypertrophic scars but is often combined with fractional laser therapy in either concurrent or alternating treatment sessions. Hypertrophic scars develop as a result of increased proliferation of dermal fibroblasts, resulting in excess of collagen in the wound, which results in an elevated cutaneous surface. Hypertrophic burn

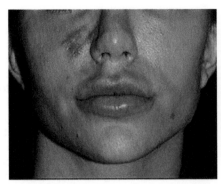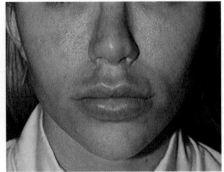

Fig. 5. Before and after early intervention 1 month postsurgical revision from traumatic injury 2 treatment sessions of pulsed dye laser, 1927, AFL.

and traumatic scars are best improved by either ablative or nonablative fractional lasers (**Fig. 6**). Ablative fractional lasers have the capacity to induce a more robust remodeling response than nonablative fractional lasers.[16,17] Ablative lasers have a significantly greater potential depth of thermal injury compared with nonablative lasers, 1.8 mm compared with 4.0 mm, respectively (LumenisS-CAAR FX software). Furthermore, tissue ablation seems to induce a modest immediate photomechanical release of tension in some restrictive scars. An appropriate degree of surrounding thermal coagulation facilitates the subsequent remodeling response. An estimation of scar pliability and thickness through palpation is central to determining appropriate laser pulse energy settings (treatment depth). Treatment depth should not exceed the thickness of the scar. Pigmentary abnormalities (hypopigmentation, hyperpigmentation, depigmentation) of scars also improve with fractional therapy.

Flat or atrophic scars from burns and trauma also respond to fractional laser therapy (**Fig. 7**). Atrophic scars are dermal depression that occur due to collagen destruction during an injury. The goal of laser treatment of atrophic scars is to stimulate collagen production within the atrophic areas. Neocollagenesis is stimulated the most from fractional laser therapy and thus makes it the best choice for flat or thin scars.

Box 2
Surgical correction of hypertrophic scars and contracture scars

Scar release with local tissue—Z-plasty, W-plasty

Scar release with skin graft

Flaps

Composite tissue allotransplantation

Autologous fat grafting

Laser therapy

PREOPERATIVE AND TREATMENT SCAR THERAPY CONSIDERATIONS

With any scar therapeutic procedure, informed consent should include a realistic discussion of therapeutic goals, limitations, and potential complications. A team approach is vital, as professional wound care, physical and occupational therapy, and surgical consultation should be available, if possible, throughout the treatment course to optimize outcomes. Pertinent historical information during the initial evaluation includes the time and mechanism of injury, surgical history and schedule of upcoming procedures, previous complications, current limitations and treatment goals, pain and sensory issues, presence of posttraumatic stress, and response to current therapy. Physical examination should elicit scar characteristics such as the presence of residual erosions and ulcers, erythema, pliability, textural irregularity, dyspigmentation, and scar thickness and degree of restriction. Associated features that may relate to adjunctive treatments include the presence or absence of residual hair, hyperhidrosis, traumatic tattoos, and related dermatologic conditions such as folliculitis.

Lastly, many patients with severe burn or traumatic scars may have developed posttraumatic stress (PTSD) and/or traumatic brain injury (TBI). If patients have either PTSD or TBI other medical paraprofessionals including psychiatrists are recommended to be part of the treatment team.

Laser-Assisted Delivery of Scars

Laser-assisted delivery uses fractional ablative columns to deliver molecules to maximize each scar treatment. These fractional ablative zones created by either CO_2 or erbium:YAG fractional lasers may be used immediately postoperatively to deliver drugs and other substances to synergistically create an enhanced therapeutic response. Ablative channels are tunable and can be

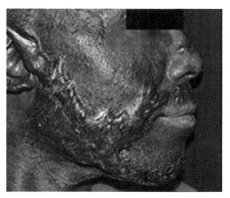 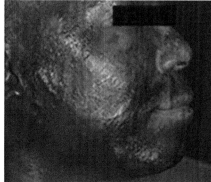

Fig. 6. Before and after hypertrophic burn scar after 5 sessions 1927 nm and 2940 AFL TAC/5FU LAD and sustained compression.

delivered in depths of 100 to 4000 μm for targeted cutaneous drug delivery. **Table 2** shows types of scars and published types of laser-assisted drug delivery. Waibel and colleagues authored a head-to-head trial looking at ways to repigment hypo-pigmentation, and the statistical winner for best repigmentation was laser-assisted delivery with bimatoprost, a prostaglandin analogue.[18] The study showed the use of the nonablative fractional laser, ablative fractional laser, ablative fractional laser with laser-assisted delivered bimatoprost, and an epidermal harvesting system. Using a fractional nonablative laser or ablative laser alone can cause repigmentation by stimulating stem cells

that exist deep along the hair follicle. Another laser often used for hypopigmentation is the 308-nm Excimer laser that will stimulate melanocytes as well in many hypopigmented scars. Initially older patients with glaucoma used drops of bimatoprost in their eyes to lower intraocular pressure and notice their eyelashes growing longer and darker. It turns out bimatoprost and other prostaglandin analogues in this drug class stimulate melanocytes to create pigmentation. The melanocytes are located in the basal laser of the epidermis and are about 90 to 100 μm in depth. In 2011 Edwards and colleagues studied the effects head-to-head on pigmentation of 3 prostaglandin

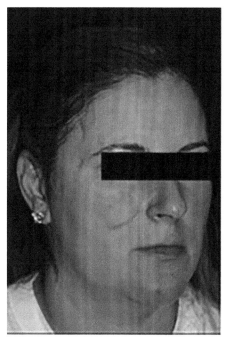 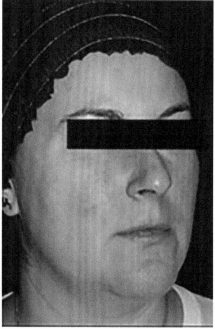

Fig. 7. Before and after dog bite atrophic trauma scar status after 6 treatment sessions of pulsed dye laser, 1550 nm nonablative fractional laser, 1927 nm nonablative thulium laser, ablative fractional laser, and poly-L-lactic acid.

Table 2
Types of scars and published types of laser-assisted drug delivery

Type of Scar	Laser-Assisted Drug	Comments
Hypertrophic scar	Corticosteroid Triamcinolone acetonide 10–40 mg/mL	Typically recommend starting with 10 mg/mL for most scars, caution in skin of color; higher doses may lead to transient or permanent damage to melanocyte/hypopigmentation
Hypertrophic scar	5-Fluoruracil	—
Atrophic scar	Poly-L-lactic acid	—
Hypopigmented scar	Poly-L-lactic acid Bimatoprost, latanoprost, and travoprost	Use twice a day after laser for 7 d

analogues including latanoprost versus bimatoprost versus travoprost on periocular skin pigmentation. The conclusions revealed that all 3 prostaglandin analogues induce darkening of the eyelid skin that is objectively detected as a decrease in the L* value. Although not reaching levels of statistical significance, this change was more dramatic for bimatoprost, more common in Caucasians and in women. The greatest degree of change occurred at 6 and 9 months after initiating treatment.[19] Lastly, a recent evidence-based practice guideline for laser-assisted drug delivery was published with pearls and pitfalls for clinicians.[20]

WHEN TO TREAT A SCAR: EARLY INTERVENTION MAKES A DIFFERENCE

Scar tissue forms slowly, and depending on which type of scar and tissue, it may take months to years. Thus, intervening early on the provider may not only mitigate but actually prevent scar formation. **Table 3** reviews early interventions that have the potential to reduce scar formation. Traditionally reconstructive efforts have been delayed until

Table 3
Early interventions that have the potential to reduce scar formation

Passive General Preventative Measures	Active Preventative Scar Mitigation
Moisturization Silicone products Sun avoidance	Contracture—stretch Raise up—compression/ pressure garments Firm—soften—massage, silicone Color/texture—laser

1 year after injury. At this time many patients have formed hypertrophic scars and have a significant decrease in range of motion. We now have clinical evidence that minimally invasive devices applied early after injury may prevent scars. After significant trauma injury fibroblasts eventually will close the wound by causing it to contract and by laying down collagen in excess. It is important to remember that hypertrophic scarring typically increases over the first 3 to 5 months after acute burn injury and can increase for over 2 years. In 2018 Karmisholt and colleagues published a systemic review on early laser intervention in different wound healing phases and potential clinical outcome on scar formation.[21] According to the results of this review, treating scars in the healing and proliferative phases decreased scar formation significantly more than the mature phase. Waibel and colleagues then performed a randomized control trial on the early intervention of fractional ablative lasers versus control for acute severe burn injuries of those hospitalized in the burn unit. This is the first randomized control study on severe trauma patients to show early intervention with the ablative fractional CO_2 laser prevents scarring when used within the first 3 months after burn injury. This information could potentially help patients live a better quality of life.[22,23] The optimal time to begin fractional laser treatment is early. As a rule, there should be a healed and intact epidermis before laser treatment. Younger, less mature scars are less tolerant of aggressive treatment and should be treated more cautiously. Mature scars, whether 1 year old or 60 years old, all respond well to laser therapy. A minimum treatment interval of 1 to 3 months between fractional laser treatments is recommended to give scar tissue, which is the compromised time to heal. Even after just one treatment session a patient may continue to have improvement for many months up to 1 year.

SUMMARY

Scar treatments have been around as long as life. The Egyptians, Romans, and Chinese all developed remedies to promote the healing of wounds to prevent scars. In these times cocoa, aloe, honey, and oak bark were used. Military medicine has challenged medicine, as our trauma surgeons can save any life and often with catastrophic injuries. We must continue to be committed through scientific inquiry to helping both wounded warriors and civilians. It is a new era in the treatment of scars. Current technologies permit successful treatment of various types of scars. The research is in an exciting state of intensive investigation, with many promising therapies being studied to evaluate their role in scar therapy. Many pharmacologic therapies may help prevent scars although more research is needed. Other scientists are studying mechanical ways to facilitate healing and prevent scarring by using methods to modulate tension vectors on skin that contribute to hypertrophic scarring. The next major breakthrough will most likely be regenerative medicine. Regenerative medicine, whether using stem cells, messenger RNA, or gene modification, may prevent scarring altogether. Current day patients receive new elegant devices such as lasers to let human body regenerate itself. Early preventative measures are emerging as an important role in scar mitigation. Laser therapy is at the forefront of treatment. Continued advances in science, medicine, and regeneration will serve to further shape the management of scars in the future.

CLINICS CARE POINTS

- Early intervention is beneficial to lessen possible complications of scarring.
- Start by evaluating the scar, noting the thickness, location, and tension forces surrounding it.
- Then, determine its phenotype for better treatment approach.
- Fractional ablative devices benefit all scar types.
- The most common corticosteroid to combine with ablative fractional lasers is triamcinolone acetonide suspension.
- When treating acne scars, treatment modalities should penetrate at least 1 mm below the skin.
- For contracture scars, z-plasties are often paired with laser treatment for best results.

SUPPLEMENTARY DATA

Supplementary data related to this article can be found online at https://doi.org/10.1016/j.fsc.2023.06.005.

REFERENCES

1. Asilian A, Darougheh A, Shariati F. New combination of triamcinolone, 5-Fluorouracil, and pulsed-dye laser for treatment of keloid and hypertrophic scars. Dermatol Surg 2006;32(7):907–15.
2. Kwan J, Wyatt M, Uebelhoer NS, et al. Functional improvement after ablative fractional laser treatment of a scar contracture. PM&R 2011;3:986–7.
3. Seago, et al. Laser treatment of traumatic scars and contractures: 2020 international consensus recommendations. Laser Surg Med 2020;52(2):96–116.
4. Waibel J, Wulkan A, Lupo M, et al. Treatment of burn scars with the 1550 nm nonablative fractional erbium laser. Laser Surg Med 2012;44:44.
5. Larson BJ, Longaker MT, Lorenz HP. Scarless fetal wound healing: a basic science review. Plast Reconstr Surg 2010;126:1172–80.
6. Einstein A. Zur Quanten Theorie der Strahlung. Physikal Zeitschr 1917;18:121–8.
7. Salameh F, Shumaker PR, Goodman GJ, et al. Energy-based devices for the treatment of Acne Scars: 2022 International consensus recommendations. Laser Surg Med 2022;54:10–26.
8. Fox L, Csongradi C, Aucamp M, et al. Treatment Modalities for Acne. Molecules 2016;21.
9. Darji K, Varade R, West D, et al. Psychosocial impact of postinflammatory hyperpigmentation in patients with acne vulgaris. J Clin Aesthet Dermatol 2017;10:18–23.
10. Sowash M, Alster T. Review of laser treatments for post-inflammatory hyperpigmentation in skin of color. Am J Clin Dermatol 2023;24(3):381–96.
11. Leclere FM, Mordon SR. Twenty-five years of active laser prevention of scars: What have we learned? J Cosmet Laser Ther 2010;12:227–34.
12. Chapas AM, Brightman L, Sukal S, et al. Successful treatment of acneiform scarring with CO2 ablative fractional resurfacing. Laser Surg Med 2008;40(6):381–6.
13. Hantash BM, Bedi VP, Kapadia B, et al. Laser Surg Med 2007;39(2):96–107.
14. Ortiz A, Elkeeb L, Truitt A, et al. Evaluation of a novel fractional resurfacing device for the treatment of acne scarring. Laser Surg Med 2009;41(2):122–7. Abstract presented at American Society for Laser Medicine and Surgery Conference, April 2008, Kissimee, FL.
15. Wang YS, Tay YK, Kwok C. Fractional ablative carbon dioxide laser in the treatment of atrophic acne scarring in Asian patients: a pilot study. J Cosmet Laser Ther 2010;12(2):61–4.

16. Jung JY, Jeong JJ, Roh HJ, et al. Early postoperative treatment of thyroidectomy scars using a fractional carbon dioxide laser. Dermatol Surg 2011;37(2): 217–23.

17. Vrijman C, van Drooge AM, Limpens J, et al. Laser and intense pulsed light therapy for the treatment of hypertrophic scars: a systematic review. Br J Dermatol 2011;165(5):934–42.

18. Waibel JS, Rudnick A, Arheart KL, et al. Re-pigmentation of hypopigmentation: fractional lasers vs laser-assisted delivery of bimatoprost vs Epidermal Melanocyte Harvesting System. J Drugs Dermatol 2019;18(11):1090–6.

19. Edwards et al. Investigative Ophthalmology & Visual Science 2011, Vol.52, 231.

20. Evidence-based clinical practice guidelines for laser-assisted drug delivery. Labadie JG, et al. JAMA Dermatol 2022. https://doi.org/10.1001/jamadermatol.2022.3234.

21. Karmisholt KE, Haerskjold A, Karlsmark T, et al. Early laser intervention to reduce scar formation – a systemic review. J Eur Acad Dermatol Venereol 2018. https://doi.org/10.1111/jdv.14856.

22. Waibel JS, Gianatasio C, Rudnick A. Randomized, controlled early intervention of dynamic mode fractional ablative CO2 laser on acute burn injuries for prevention of pathological scarring. Lasers Surg Med 2020;52(2):117–24.

23. Petro JA. An idiosyncratic history of burn scars. Semin Cutan Med Surg 2015;34(1):2–6.

Ablative Laser Therapy of Skin

J. Kevin Duplechain, MD

KEYWORDS

- Ablative laser therapy • Thermal relaxation time of skin • Fully ablative resurfacing
- Fractional resurfacing • Carbon dioxide resurfacing • Chromophore

KEY POINTS

- Skin rejuvenation continues to be one of the most popular requested cosmetic procedures.
- Ablative lasers vaporize the tissue, removing all or part of the skin surface in the treatment area. The damaged skin undergoes healing processes and is replaced with healthy tissue.
- The most common indications for both full-field and fractional laser resurfacing are superficial dyschromias, dermatoheliosis, textural anomalies, superficial to deep rhytids, acne scars, and surgical scars.
- Using treatment parameters that combine depth of injury, energy of ablation, and density can provide safe and reliable treatments and consistent outcomes.
- Treatment should be tailored according to each patient's specific needs, skin characteristics, and treatment area.

 Video content accompanies this article at http://www.facialplastic.theclinics.com.

INTRODUCTION

Ablative laser skin resurfacing is used for removing superficial dermal layers of the skin to reduce cutaneous signs of photoaging as well as for treatment of facial wrinkles, acne and surgical scars, traumatic scars, and numerous types of superficial skin lesions, and to enhance the effects of facial plastic surgery, such as facelift and blepharoplasty.

History of the Development of Ablative Lasers for Skin Therapy

Continuous-wave carbon dioxide (CO_2) lasers for skin resurfacing were introduced in the 1980s, gaining popularity and often replacing chemical peels and dermabrasion. The 10,600-nm CO_2 laser wavelength is absorbed by its primary chromophore, water, which is heated, vaporizing the tissue and removing the entire skin surface in the treatment area. The depth of injury is determined by the

energy level applied. At the time of its introduction into clinical use, resurfacing using the CO_2 laser required high operator skill due to pulse width and power constraints. Continuous-wave devices could either be used at high power, which caused less thermal damage but vaporization depth was difficult to control due to the need to sweep over the skin swiftly and uniformly, or at low power, which helped control penetration depth but could cause excessive thermal damage. As a result, the extent of tissue destruction was unpredictable and was associated with unacceptable risks of impaired wound healing and scarring.[1–3]

In an attempt to minimize complications, short-pulse laser devices were developed, which exposed the tissue to less than 1 msec of laser energy at a time, allowing tissue ablation with limited residual thermal damage of approximately 75 to 100 μm. Despite excellent improvement of wrinkle appearance and skin laxity tightening within a

Division of Facial Plastic Surgery, Department of Otolaryngology, Tulane Medical School, 1103 Kaliste Saloom Road, Suite 300, Lafayette, 70508, LA, USA
E-mail address: jkdmd@drduplechain.com

Facial Plast Surg Clin N Am 31 (2023) 463–473
https://doi.org/10.1016/j.fsc.2023.05.002
1064-7406/23/© 2023 Elsevier Inc. All rights reserved.

short period of time, this technology was associated with significant downtime as well as long-term hypopigmentation in a large proportion of patients.[4]

The erbium-doped yttrium aluminum garnet (Er:YAG) laser, which delivers energy at 2940 nm was introduced at the turn of the century. As 2940 nm is at the peak of water absorption, vaporization is the primary mode of action, whereas coagulation is minimal and diffusion of heat to surrounding tissue is greatly reduced, lowering the risk of scarring and damage to pilosebaceous units.[5] The delivered energy density (fluence) of the Er:YAG laser is linearly correlated with the depth of tissue ablated, with 3 to 4 μm of tissue removed per J/cm^2; thus, multiple passes can be used to produce deeper tissue removal without additive residual thermal injury. As a result, the recovery time to full epithelialization after deep full-field Er:YAG laser resurfacing is 7 to 10 days followed by 3 to 6 weeks of erythema. Comparative studies have shown that the combined depth of ablation and coagulation determined the length of recovery following the use of Er:YAG lasers.[6,7] Variable or long-pulse Er:YAG lasers enable controlling the amount of residual thermal injury produced for a given amount of tissue removal. Comparison of Er:YAG to CO_2 resurfacing showed more long-term wound contraction and fibroplasia with CO_2 treatments.[8]

Additional advances in skin resurfacing techniques occurred with the introduction of fractional photothermolysis technology, whereby the laser beam is manipulated through a diffractive lens, creating multiple microscopic laser beams. Each microscopic laser energy beam creates small columns (< 400 μm in diameter) of thermal damage, called microscopic thermal zones (MTZs), whose penetration depth is proportional to the laser energy emitted. Fractionating the pulsed ablative laser energy that covers only a fraction of the treated area (approximately 5%–30%) enables rapid reepithelialization from the undamaged, adjacent epidermis separating the MTZs, facilitating repair and remodeling of the epidermis and dermis.[9] Histologically, the MTZ of ablative fractionated laser comprise a central column of stratum corneum, epidermal, and dermal ablation lined by a thin eschar and surrounded by an annular coagulation zone (penumbra).[10,11] In contrast to full-field resurfacing whereby healing occurs from deep structures only, healing following ablative fractional photothermolysis occurs from adjacent structures as well as from deeper structures. This less destructive technology further reduced the incidence of adverse events and increased the degree of therapeutic control[12]; however, multiple treatments were required and the clinical response was more limited compared with full-field ablative resurfacing.[11,13]

As ablative lasers vaporize tissue, their effect is more "destructive" with longer downtime and recovery compared with nonablative lasers that leave the skin intact. Nevertheless, they result in better improvements when treating severe facial wrinkles, dyspigmentation, and textural skin.

Depending on the indication, the technician may choose to use a specific ablative laser (eg, CO_2 or Er:YAG) with a multitude of different settings, including fractional versus nonfractional, to achieve the desired result and, more importantly, minimize laser-associated complications such as scarring, persistent erythema, and dyspigmentation.

Patient Selection

Careful patient selection and knowledge of potential complications are essential for achieving consistent results. The initial consultation should begin with an evaluation of the patient's ethnicity, skin type, and degree of photodamage. Darker skin types (IV–VI) have increased epidermal melanin, larger and more widely distributed melanosomes, and reactive fibroblasts,[14] which result in a tendency for hyperpigmentation in response to light stimuli or trauma.[15] The characteristics of photoaging differ by ethnicity. For example, photoaging in Asian individuals is characterized by pigmentary alterations, lentigines, and seborrheic keratoses rather than fine lines and deep rhytids observed in Caucasian individuals.[16,17]

Understanding patients' expectations in an esthetic treatment is crucial. For example, ablative laser resurfacing may be used for improving tone, texture, and wrinkles but it is not a substitute for a facelift or a necklift. During the initial consult, the treating physician should discuss healing times and the return to social and work-related activities. These timelines will affect the type and intensity of the treatment rendered.

The most common indications for both full-field and fractional laser resurfacing are superficial dyschromias, dermatoheliosis, textural anomalies, superficial to deep rhytids, acne scars, and surgical scars. Other conditions that may respond favorably include rhinophyma, sebaceous hyperplasia, xanthelasma, syringomas, actinic cheilitis, and diffuse actinic keratoses. Dyschromias such as melasma have been successfully treated with fractional resurfacing but results are not consistent. Better treatments for melasma currently exist, particularly with the advent and use of tranexamic acid accompanied by nonablative neodymium-doped YAG laser treatments.

Pretreatment Considerations

Herpes simplex virus 1 reactivation may occur in patients undergoing ablative facial laser resurfacing and may delay healing and result in severe scarring[18]; therefore, antivirals should be prescribed to every patient.[19–21]

Ablative resurfacing can produce a myriad of wounds from very superficial epidermal injuries to deeper dermal wounds. The extent of the wound healing period and the final cosmetic outcome depend on the preoperative and post-resurfacing care regimes.[22] Bacterial infection after laser skin resurfacing may affect healing by increasing the depth of the original wound and delaying reepithelialization, consequently increasing the risk of persistent erythema, dyschromias, and scarring.[23] Infections are sometimes noticeable only in the second week after the procedure.[24] Infectious agents identified following laser resurfacing procedures were similar to those reported for burn injuries, including *Pseudomonas aeruginosa, Staphylococcus aureus, Staphylococcus epidermis, and Staphylococcus aureus.*[25,26] Prophylactic oral antibiotics should be prescribed to prevent secondary bacterial infection.[23] Oral antibiotics should be started 1 day before the procedure and be continued until reepithelialization has been completed.[20,21,24]

Although it is debated whether pretreatment with topical bleaching agents, such as hydroquinone cream, reduce the risk of post-inflammatory hyperpigmentation after laser resurfacing,[27,28] this has been shown in darker skin types, especially after laser resurfacing.[28]

Patients who were exposed to the sun or actively tanned should wait until the tan fades (2–4 weeks) before starting ablative laser therapy.[29]

Posttreatment

Treatment with any ablative laser system involves a healing phase that usually lasts 5 to 10 days.

The lack of postablative laser treatment protocols was responsible to some degree for the demise of ablative CO_2 use in the 1990s. Posttreatment care should be diligent and the physician must be involved in all of its care aspects.

Application of topical corticosteroids immediately after ablative skin resurfacing treatment has been shown to effectively decrease post-inflammatory hyperpigmentation, especially in individuals with dark skin types.[30] The persistent use of corticosteroids may however significantly reduce the expression of messenger RNA and significantly reduce the amount of collagen regeneration postprocedure.[31] Mineral sunblocks that contain titanium dioxide or zinc oxide prevent potential sensitization effects associated with the use of chemical sunscreens.[32,33] Topical skin bleachers/lighteners, such as ascorbic, tranexamic, glycolic and kojic acids, and hydroquinone, may be used for treating hyperpigmentation after erythema has subsided.[22,34,35]

Thermal damage may cause localized immunosuppression that may lead to a secondary infection.[36] The use of topical antibiotics to prevent infection during wound healing is limited by the risk of contact dermatitis in laser-abraded skin.[4,20,23,37]

Antivirals should continue to be used after the treatment to prevent herpes simplex virus 1 reactivation.[19–21]

I currently use a formulated perfluorodecalin product which has been shown to accelerate wound healing and significantly reduce postprocedure complications including persistent erythema, acneiform eruptions, and delayed healing.[38]

Treatment Parameters

When planning an ablative resurfacing treatment for any area of the body, three factors must be considered: energy used, density, and the pulsed duration of the laser. As skin depth differs throughout the face and body, it is imperative to consider skin depth when selecting the appropriate energy level. New technology lasers, such as the Lumenis Alpha UltraPulse, now provide depth of injury parameters as energy levels are selected. The density must also be adjusted according to the treatment area and the depth of injury. Fully ablative treatments remove the entire surface area of the treated zone. The wound or depth of injury can be very superficial, affecting the epidermis only, or it can reach papillary or reticular dermal elements. Deeper penetration into the reticular dermis must be fractionated and should be reserved for facial treatments. Creating an injury that extends into the reticular dermis in non-facial areas has been shown to significantly increase the risk of scarring (**Fig. 1**). The pulsed duration of the laser must also be considered. The thermal relaxation time (TRT) of skin is approximately 8 msec.[39] The ability to lase and successfully ablate skin within the TRT significantly reduces the risk of additional coagulation, thereby preventing the enlargement of the laser ablation wound, which essentially affects the density of the rendered treatment. Longer pulsed lasers that mimic the early scanner type devices are known to create wounds with significantly longer wound healing times and increased complications. The primary reason for this phenomenon is the time on tissue or pulse width.

I have been using the UltraPulse CO_2 Laser System (Lumenis BE, Yokne'am, Israel) since 2008.

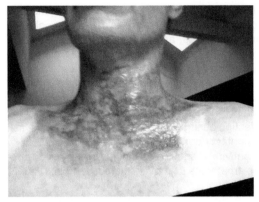

Fig. 1. Penetration into the reticular dermis in non-facial areas has been shown to significantly increase the risk of scarring. The photo depicts a neck 7 days after fractional erbium resurfacing.

The settings described below reflect my experience with this device.

Periorbital Treatment

Changes around the eyes are often among the first perceived signs of facial aging. Fractional CO_2 laser treatment is a useful noninvasive alternative to blepharoplasty for reestablishing a more youthful appearance. In addition, it is a valuable adjunct to blepharoplasty to improve the textural changes associated with aging.

Common treatment parameters for this area include a fractionated treatment around the lateral canthal area at an injury depth of approximately 550 μm using energy of 15 mJ and 20% density. The DeepFX scanner (Lumenis) is set to a density of 10%, and two passes are completed. Recent advances with a randomized deep mode have demonstrated the ability to increase density to approximately 20% in a single pass without significant changes in healing. The area is then treated with the superficial Active FX scanner (Lumenis) at 80 mJ with a density of approximately 50%. The laser must not be used to treat the area below the supratarsal fold on the eyelid. In addition, metal eye shields should be used in all cases of facial skin resurfacing. At these settings, the depth of injury using the superficial scanner reaches the papillary dermis of the eyelid skin. Decreasing the density has proven to minimize the risk of scarring or ectropion related to resurfacing.[40,41] I have found no occurrences of delayed healing or ectropion with these parameters.

Treatment benefits include improvement or disappearance of mild to moderate rhytids, improved skin texture and tone, decreased pore size, and improvement and reduction in skin laxity (**Fig. 2**)

Perioral Treatment

The perioral area often requires a more aggressive treatment. Because the epidermis and papillary dermis in the perioral area approach a depth of 250 μm,[42] higher energy settings may be safely used. Commonly, a deep scanner is used at a density of 15% and energy of 17.5 mJ to reach a depth of 600 μm. With this setting, two passes may be safely performed. Once completed, the superficial scanner may be used at 100 to 125 mJ with a density setting of 80%. This will essentially remove all of the epidermal and some papillary dermal components, resulting in a deeper injury consistent with a second-degree burn. This more aggressive treatment will require approximately 10 days to heal (**Fig. 3**).

Hand Rejuvenation

Rejuvenation of the hands continues to be an interest of many patients. Ablative laser treatment combined with a filler, such as fat or calcium hydroxylapatite, can significantly improve the appearance of the hands. Typically, the dorsal area of the hands is prepared for a sterile injection technique. A small amount of local anesthesia is placed between the four knuckles. A 25-gauge cannula is used for injecting the calcium hydroxylapatite, whereas a 19 gauge cannula is used for injecting fat. To provide additional comfort, a small amount of lidocaine is mixed with the fat before injection. Once the injection is completed, the hands are superficially lasered at a power setting of 80 mJ and 50% density. The healing process usually takes about 2 weeks, with few limitations. The laser power settings typically cause minimal crusting, and most patients find recovery simple.

Neck Rejuvenation

The aging neck is characterized by lipodystrophy, platysmal bands, and jowls that extend into the neck.[43] As jowls develop, the chin and jawline lose definition and horizontal and radial necklines become more noticeable.[44] Like the face, the neck is subject to photodamage.[45] Patients who seek facial rejuvenation often request a neck treatment to ensure a homogenous and completely rejuvenated face and neck.

The use of CO_2 laser for neck skin rejuvenation has been described in several studies.[46–49] Reports of scarring have raised concerns about deep neck treatments.[50,51]

Before starting neck skin rejuvenation, it is crucial that the expectations of both the surgeon and patient are aligned. It is important to understand that aggressive deep neck treatments are

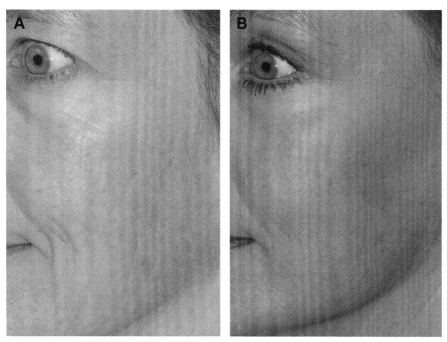

Fig. 2. A female patient (*A*) before and (*B*) 3 months after undergoing blepharoplasty and facelift with combined deep and superficial CO_2 resurfacing. Note the significant improvement in the quality of the skin.

not a replacement for neck and facelift surgery and therefore should not be performed. Attempts to injure the platysma muscle to elevate and tighten it should not be performed with an ablative laser. The key components of the neck skin should be considered when planning treatment. Beyond the first cervical crease, the neck skin is deplete of

skin adnexal structures; therefore, laser treatment parameters must be modified significantly to safely treat this area. The skin above the first cervical crease is more similar histologically to facial skin, and settings can be similar to those used for treating facial skin along the jawline. During facelift and necklift surgery, the neck is treated to

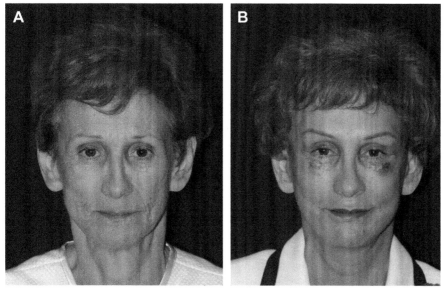

Fig. 3. A 74-year-old patient (*A*) before and (*B*) 11 days after undergoing a facelift and fat grafting with combined deep and superficial CO_2 resurfacing. The early result at 11 days indicates acceptable healing times even with combined therapy.

improve the overall skin texture, but additional tightening is usually not performed. Completely undermined neck skin may be treated safely with ablative CO_2 laser using the UltraPulse device at an energy setting of 80 mJ, with a density of 50% and a frequency of 250 Hz.

Treatment of Scars

Ablative fractional CO_2 laser is currently considered the gold standard treatment for hypertrophic scarring. The use of the CO_2 laser for treatment of facial acne scarring was reported in four studies. In a study on 25 patients aged 17 to 62 years, patients demonstrated overall improvement of acne scarring with significantly greater degrees of improvement in the forehead, perioral region, and medial cheek compared with the temple and lateral cheek. There were no cases of prolonged hyperpigmentation or erythema persisting beyond 3 months and no long-term complications were reported.[52] Histologic examination of skin biopsy specimens from nine patients (age range, 25–41 years, Fitzpatrick skin types I–IV) taken immediately after treatment with the CO_2 laser showed full-thickness loss of epidermis with formation of a homogeneous hypereosinophilic zone of thermal damage in the papillary dermis, extending focally into the reticular dermis. Skin biopsy specimens taken after 3 months showed a thick band of papillary dermal fibrosis in skin treated with the CO_2 laser.[53] Vaporization depth and residual thermal damage following use of the "superficial" or "deep" scanning modes of the 40 W continuous-wave CO_2 laser was similar in biopsies taken from 14 patients aged 24 to 54 years with Fitzpatrick skin type I–IV.[54] Moderate to severe acne scars significantly improved following treatment with the CO_2 laser using a "double-layer" technique.[55] Varying degrees of pain, erythema, edema, oozing of blood, and exudate were observed immediately after each treatment. Two cases (10%) of persistent erythema were reported which lasted for 2 to 3 days and two cases (10%) of hyperpigmentation which lasted 3 to 5 days. Average downtime was 6 days.

The use of the CO_2 laser was found to be a highly effective therapy for management of the persistent, scarred, and sinus tract lesions of hidradenitis suppurativa.[56,57] Madan and colleagues[57] reported on CO_2 laser treatment of recalcitrant hidradenitis suppurativa in nine patients aged 27 to 52 years who had failed to improve on medical and other surgical treatments. Mean wound healing time was 2 weeks (range 1–4). Good clinical results, evidenced by absence of active discharging lesions at the treatment sites, were seen in seven patients with no recurrence at 12-month of follow-up. Six patients reported that their hidradenitis suppurativa was inactive 12 months after the laser treatment. Two patients still had active hidradenitis suppurativa at untreated sites adjacent to treated sites within the anatomical unit. One patient developed discharging lesions at treated sites 3 months after surgery. Further laser treatment at this site was effective in achieving remission. Seven patients were able to discontinue all systemic treatments without relapse. Scar contracture not restricting limb mobility was noted in two patients. Hazen and Hazen[56] reported on treatment of 61 patients aged 21 to 73 years. Following treatment with the CO_2 laser, all patients healed with cosmetic and comfort qualities deemed acceptable to excellent in all areas. There were no instances of reduced range of motion. Follow-up after treatment noted an average of 4.1 years without disease recurrence in treated areas (range 1–17 years).

Acikel and colleagues[58] investigated the effectiveness of CO_2 laser resurfacing and thin skin grafting in camouflaging self-inflicted razor blade incision scars in the upper arm, forearm, and anterior chest of 16 white male patients aged 16 to 41 years. All of the procedures were successful, and the postoperative course was uneventful for all of the patients. Skin graft donor sites healed in 5 to 7 days. Hair growth through the skin graft was excellent, and normal hair patterns were regained over the treatment sites. Eighty percent of the existing hypertrophic scars were totally resolved after the operation; 20% of hypertrophic scars showed a tendency to recur and responded well to repetitive intralesional steroid injections and silicone gel sheeting. Complications included partial graft loss on the anterior chest caused by inadequate immobilization was observed in one patient and the wound reepithelialized spontaneously. Significant hyperpigmentation developed in one patient who did not protect the grafted area from sunlight. Small inclusion cysts were observed in five patients in the early postoperative period, which were treated by opening the top of the cyst and removing the contents.

Du and colleagues[59] reported apparent esthetic scar improvement following CO_2 laser treatment before skin suture during scar revision surgery in 10 patients aged 22 to 47 years with Fitzpatrick skin types III–IV. Erythema was resolved within 3 months in all of the cases. No cases of permanent hyperpigmentation, hypopigmentation, or scar hyperplasia were observed.

Zhang and colleagues[60] compared the outcomes of treatment of fresh surgical scars longer than 2 cm in the neck and face with CO_2 laser to the outcomes of untreated surgical scars. All 18 patients in the treatment group had significant improvements in their surgical scars after the laser therapy. Assessments from both patients and physicians were highly consistent. The overall effective rate was 100%, with excellent responses in 16 patients (88.9%) and good responses in two patients (11.1%). The most significant improvements were color, vascularity, and hardness, which all reached statistically significant differences before and after the treatment. Untreated scars improved statistically significant less than the CO_2-treated scars.

Combined Surgical and Ablative CO_2 Laser Treatments as an Adjunct to Facelift

The ability to safely resurface skin during facelift surgery is a key component of successful facial rejuvenation. For many years, it was considered unsafe to perform laser skin ablation on undermined skin during facelift/necklift. The procedures were commonly staged, and patients were treated later, after the facelift had healed, or areas of undermined skin were not treated. Chemical peels were often used in the perioral area, but not elsewhere. I performed 35% trichloroacetic acid peels during facelift surgery for some time, and although no scarring occurred, the results were inconsistent probably due to being cautious not to over penetrate the skin with the peeling solution. With the advent of more precise ablative laser technology, I began to use laser resurfacing in patients undergoing facelifts in 2008. The results of combined skin rejuvenation and facelift were dramatic, as the "canvas" had been completely rejuvenated as well. Currently, deep plan facelift is performed in my practice, but I do elevate a skin flap of approximately 5 to 6 cm before entering the deep plane. The areas over the deep plane and the more superficial skin-only flap are lased using the same settings. I have not encountered skin loss in these areas with over 1500 cases of combined facelift and laser skin

ablation. Treatment parameters are typically 90 to 100 mJ with 70% to 80% density. The neck is commonly treated as using energy of 70 to 80 mJ with 50% density.

The simultaneous treatment of facelift and ablative laser skin rejuvenation significantly improves the final results of facial rejuvenation. Patients are extremely satisfied with the adjunctive procedure, and do not find the healing time of 1 week a significant issue. The UltraPulse device used by the author possesses a coherent beam. Coupled with the ultra-short pulse duration, a painting technique is used to reach the desired density without creating any stamping or true delineation of lased and non-lased skin. The attached video demonstrates this technique (Video 1)

Case study 1
A 54-year-old patient had extensive weight loss over 18 months and chose to have facial rejuvenation. She was interested in having a natural look and wanted to see some improvement in her photoaged skin. She underwent an endoscopic brow lift, upper and lower lid blepharoplasty, and a deep-plane facelift. Fat grafting was also performed as well as a full face and neck CO_2 resurfacing procedure. CO_2 treatment settings were 100 mJ at a density of 80% and a frequency of 250 Hz (**Fig. 4**).

Case study 2
A 52-year-old patient with extensive sun exposure was seen in consultation for facial rejuvenation. Her extensive sun exposure and long history of smoking presented several concerns regarding treatment, including the simultaneous use of laser resurfacing during a surgical procedure. The patient underwent an endoscopic brow lift, facelift, upper and lower blepharoplasty, fat grafting, and full face and neck laser resurfacing with the CO_2 laser (settings: energy 90 mJ, 90% density, frequency 250 Hz, depth of injury approximately 80 μm).

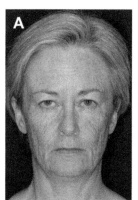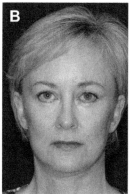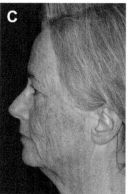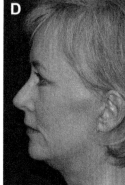

Fig. 4. Frontal view before (*A*) and 1 month after surgery (*B*). Lateral view before (*C*) and 1 month after surgery (*D*).

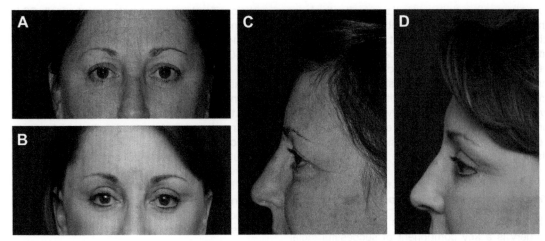

Fig. 5. Frontal view before (*A*) and 3 months after surgery (*B*). Lateral view before (*C*) and 3 months after surgery (*D*).

Although her face healed without complications, she did have a small amount of skin loss in the post-auricular area which was not lased (**Fig. 5**).

Case study 3

A 74-year-old patient requested to treat her smoker's lines in the perioral area. She also requested complete facial rejuvenation, including an endoscopic brow lift, facelift, upper and lower blepharoplasty, and full-face skin resurfacing. The perioral area was treated with 125 mJ, 100% density, and a frequency of 250 Hz. Once the

eschar was removed, a second pass was performed at 80 mJ, 50% density, and 250 Hz (**Fig. 6**).

DISCUSSION

Ablative laser skin resurfacing is a very powerful treatment of patients who desire an improvement in the quality of their skin. As a stand-alone procedure, it can significantly improve fine wrinkles, pigmentation issues, and actinic keratosis. When used in conjunction with deep fractional resurfacing, volumetric reduction may occur, which can reduce the general surface area of the treatment area

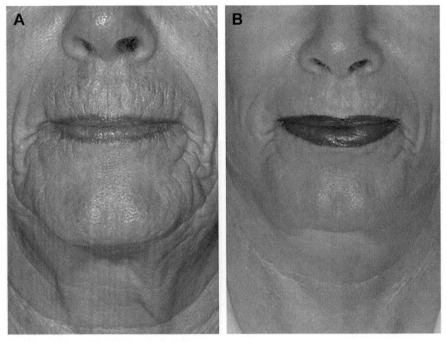

Fig. 6. Frontal view before (*A*) and 3 months after surgery (*B*).

and decrease the apparent laxity. When used in conjunction with a surgical procedure such as facelift, skin rejuvenation includes additional tightening and collagen restoration along with a completely fresh "canvas." These outcomes provide a significant benefit and joy to the patient's experience.

Skin resurfacing relies on the laser device to provide safe ablation and coagulation in a finite period to prevent overheating and over-ablation or coagulation. Longer duration treatments outside the TRT of skin account for unsuspected complications such as burns or an extremely long healing duration. Many devices are suitable for skin resurfacing, but the physician must be provided with complete information (eg, treatment settings, how to correctly operate the device and its handpieces or scanners, how to avoid complications) to achieve a successful treatment.

Treatment should be tailored according to each patient's specific needs, skin characteristics, and treatment area. These parameters (eg, energy levels, treatment density, and frequency) must be noted in the patient's record. When necessary, changes within the treatment protocol for different treatment areas should also be noted in the patient record. Simply stating that laser resurfacing was performed is an incomplete record and provides room for significant scrutiny if complications were to occur.

Safe and effective laser skin resurfacing should be considered in most patients undergoing facial rejuvenation. The benefits significantly outweigh the associated risk when performed appropriately.

CLINICS CARE POINTS

- Careful patient selection and knowledge of potential complications are essential for achieving consistent results.
- Understanding patients' expectations in an esthetic treatment is crucial.
- Treatment should be tailored according to each patient's specific needs, skin characteristics, and treatment area.
- Posttreatment care should be diligent and the physician must be involved in all of its care aspects.
- The simultaneous treatment of facelift and ablative laser skin rejuvenation significantly improves the final results of facial rejuvenation.
- Learn all that you can about the laser you use and use it every day to perfect your treatment protocols.

DISCLOSURE

J.K. Duplechain is a member of the Speakers' bureau of Lumenis and Apyx Medical and reports ownership of Cutagenesis stock options.

SUPPLEMENTARY DATA

Supplementary data related to this article can be found online at https://doi.org/10.1016/j.fsc.2023.05.002.

REFERENCES

1. David L, Lask G, Glassberg E, et al. Laser abrasion for cosmetic and medical treatment of facial actinic damage. Cutis 1989;43(6):583–7.
2. Fitzpatrick RE, Goldman MP. Advances in carbon dioxide laser surgery. Clin Dermatol 1995;13(1):35–47.
3. Hobbs ER, Bailin PL, Wheeland RG, et al. Superpulsed lasers: minimizing thermal damage with short duration, high irradiance pulses. J Dermatol Surg Oncol 1987;13(9):955–64.
4. Weinstein C, Pozner JN, Ramirez OM. Complications of carbon dioxide laser resurfacing and their prevention. Aesthet Surg J 1997;17(4):216–25.
5. Bass LS. Erbium:YAG laser skin resurfacing: preliminary clinical evaluation. Ann Plast Surg 1998;40(4):328–34.
6. Pozner JM, Goldberg DJ. Histologic effect of a variable pulsed Er:YAG laser. Dermatol Surg 2000;26(8):733–6.
7. Pozner JN, Roberts TL 3rd. Variable-pulse width ER:YAG laser resurfacing. Clin Plast Surg 2000;27(2):263–71, xi.
8. Ross EV, McKinlay JR, Anderson RR. Why does carbon dioxide resurfacing work? A review. Arch Dermatol 1999;135(4):444–54.
9. Hantash BM, Bedi VP, Chan KF, et al. Ex vivo histological characterization of a novel ablative fractional resurfacing device. Lasers Surg Med 2007;39(2):87–95.
10. Hantash BM, Bedi VP, Kapadia B, et al. In vivo histological evaluation of a novel ablative fractional resurfacing device. Lasers Surg Med 2007;39(2):96–107.
11. Geronemus RG. Fractional photothermolysis: current and future applications. Lasers Surg Med 2006;38(3):169–76.
12. Manstein D, Herron GS, Sink RK, et al. Fractional photothermolysis: a new concept for cutaneous remodeling using microscopic patterns of thermal injury. Lasers Surg Med 2004;34(5):426–38.
13. Laubach HJ, Tannous Z, Anderson RR, et al. Skin responses to fractional photothermolysis. Lasers Surg Med 2006;38(2):142–9.
14. Alexis AF. Lasers and light-based therapies in ethnic skin: treatment options and recommendations for

Fitzpatrick skin types V and VI. Br J Dermatol 2013; 169(Suppl 3):91–7.

15. Wat H, Wu DC, Chan HH. Fractional resurfacing in the Asian patient: Current state of the art. Lasers Surg Med 2017;49(1):45–59.

16. Nouveau-Richard S, Yang Z, Mac-Mary S, et al. Skin ageing: a comparison between Chinese and European populations. A pilot study. J Dermatol Sci 2005;40(3):187–93.

17. Tsukahara K, Fujimura T, Yoshida Y, et al. Comparison of age-related changes in wrinkling and sagging of the skin in Caucasian females and in Japanese females. J Cosmet Sci 2004;55(4):351–71.

18. Bisaccia E, Scarborough D. Herpes simplex virus prophylaxis with famciclovir in patients undergoing aesthetic facial CO2 laser resurfacing. Cutis 2003; 72(4):327–8.

19. Nestor MS. Prophylaxis for and treatment of uncomplicated skin and skin structure infections in laser and cosmetic surgery. J Drugs Dermatol 2005;4(6 Suppl):s20–5.

20. Lowe NJ, Lask G, Griffin ME. Laser skin resurfacing. Pre- and posttreatment guidelines. Dermatol Surg 1995;21(12):1017–9.

21. Tanzi EL, Lupton JR, Alster TS. Lasers in dermatology: four decades of progress. J Am Acad Dermatol 2003;49(1):1–31 [quiz: 31-34].

22. Duke D, Grevelink JM. Care before and after laser skin resurfacing. A survey and review of the literature. Dermatol Surg 1998;24(2):201–6.

23. Ross EV, Amesbury EC, Barile A, et al. Incidence of postoperative infection or positive culture after facial laser resurfacing: a pilot study, a case report, and a proposal for a rational approach to antibiotic prophylaxis. J Am Acad Dermatol 1998;39(6):975–81.

24. Manuskiatti W, Fitzpatrick RE, Goldman MP, et al. Prophylactic antibiotics in patients undergoing laser resurfacing of the skin. J Am Acad Dermatol 1999; 40(1):77–84.

25. Sriprachya-Anunt S, Fitzpatrick RE, Goldman MP, et al. Infections complicating pulsed carbon dioxide laser resurfacing for photoaged facial skin. Dermatol Surg 1997;23(7):527–35 [discussion: 535-526].

26. Phillips LG, Heggers JP, Robson MC, et al. The effect of endogenous skin bacteria on burn wound infection. Ann Plast Surg 1989;23(1):35–8.

27. West TB, Alster TS. Effect of pretreatment on the incidence of hyperpigmentation following cutaneous CO2 laser resurfacing. Dermatol Surg 1999;25(1):15–7.

28. Alajlan AM, Alsuwaidan SN. Acne scars in ethnic skin treated with both non-ablative fractional 1,550 nm and ablative fractional CO2 lasers: comparative retrospective analysis with recommended guidelines. Lasers Surg Med 2011;43(8):787–91.

29. Alster TS, Li MK. Dermatologic Laser Side Effects and Complications: Prevention and Management. Am J Clin Dermatol 2020;21(5):711–23.

30. Cheyasak N, Manuskiatti W, Maneeprasopchoke P, et al. Topical corticosteroids minimise the risk of postinflammatory hyper-pigmentation after ablative fractional CO2 laser resurfacing in Asians. Acta Derm Venereol 2015;95(2):201–5.

31. Nuutinen P, Riekki R, Parikka M, et al. Modulation of collagen synthesis and mRNA by continuous and intermittent use of topical hydrocortisone in human skin. Br J Dermatol 2003;148(1):39–45.

32. Wanitphakdeedecha R, Phuardchantuk R, Manuskiatti W. The use of sunscreen starting on the first day after ablative fractional skin resurfacing. J Eur Acad Dermatol Venereol 2014;28(11):1522–8.

33. Boonchai W, Sathaworawong A, Wongpraparut C, et al. The sensitization potential of sunscreen after ablative fractional skin resurfacing using modified human repeated insult patch test. J Dermatol Treat 2015;26(5):485–8.

34. Alster TS, Khoury RR. Treatment of laser complications. Facial Plast Surg 2009;25(5):316–23.

35. Alster TS, Lupton JR. Prevention and treatment of side effects and complications of cutaneous laser resurfacing. Plast Reconstr Surg 2002;109(1): 308–16 [discussion: 317-308].

36. Munster AM. Immunologic response of trauma and burns. An overview. Am J Med 1984;76(3a):142–5.

37. Waldorf HA, Kauvar AN, Geronemus RG. Skin resurfacing of fine to deep rhytides using a char-free carbon dioxide laser in 47 patients. Dermatol Surg 1995;21(11):940–6.

38. Duplechain JK, Rubin MG, Kim K. Novel posttreatment care after ablative and fractional CO2 laser resurfacing. J Cosmet Laser Ther 2014;16(2):77–82.

39. Anderson RR, Parrish JA. Selective photothermolysis: precise microsurgery by selective absorption of pulsed radiation. Science 1983;220(4596):524–7.

40. Mezzana P, Scarinci F, Costantino A, et al. Lower eyelid ablative fractional resurfacing: a new technique to treat skin laxity and photoaging. Acta Chir Plast 2010;52(2–4):35–8.

41. Özkoca D, Aşkın Ö, Engin B. Treatment of periorbital and perioral wrinkles with fractional Er:YAG laser: What are the effects of age, smoking, and Glogau stage? J Cosmet Dermatol 2021;20(9):2800–4.

42. Sasaki GH, Travis HM, Tucker B. Fractional CO2 laser resurfacing of photoaged facial and nonfacial skin: histologic and clinical results and side effects. J Cosmet Laser Ther 2009;11(4):190–201.

43. Rohrich RJ, Rios JL, Smith PD, et al. Neck Rejuvenation Revisited. Plast Reconstr Surg 2006;118(5): 1251–63.

44. Brandt FS, Boker A. Botulinum toxin for the treatment of neck lines and neck bands. Dermatol Clin 2004; 22(2):159–66.

45. Goldman MP, Fitzpatrick RE, Manuskiatti W. Laser resurfacing of the neck with the Erbium:YAG laser. Dermatol Surg 1999;25(3):164–8.

46. Fanous N, Prinja N, Sawaf M. Laser resurfacing of the neck: A review of 48 cases. Aesthetic Plast Surg 1998;22(3):173–9.

47. Behroozan DS, Christian MM, Moy RL. Short-pulse carbon dioxide laser resurfacing of the neck. J Am Acad Dermatol 2000;43(Part 1):72–6.

48. Fitzpatrick RE, Goldman MP, Sriprachya-Anunt S. Resurfacing of photodamaged skin on the neck with an UltraPulse® carbon dioxide laser. Laser Surg Med 2001;28(2):145–9.

49. Kilmer SL, Chotzen V, Zelickson BD, et al. Full-face laser resurfacing using a supplemented topical anesthesia protocol. Arch Dermatol 2003;139(10):1279–83.

50. Avram MM, Tope WD, Yu T, et al. Hypertrophic scarring of the neck following ablative fractional carbon dioxide laser resurfacing. Lasers Surg Med 2009;41(3):185–8.

51. Duplechain JK. Severe neck scarring: A consequence of fractional CO2 laser resurfacing. J Cosmet Laser Ther 2016;18(6):352–4.

52. Trimas SJ, Boudreaux CE, Metz RD. Carbon dioxide laser abrasion. Is it appropriate for all regions of the face? Arch Facial Plast Surg 2000;2(2):137–40.

53. Acland KM, Calonje E, Seed PT, et al. A clinical and histologic comparison of electrosurgical and carbon dioxide laser peels. J Am Acad Dermatol 2001;44(3):492–6.

54. Huilgol SC, Poon E, Calonje E, et al. Scanned continuous wave CO2 laser resurfacing: a closer look at the different scanning modes. Dermatol Surg 2001;27(5):467–70.

55. Yang Z, Jiang S, Zhang Y, et al. Self-contrast study of pinprick therapy combined with super pulse fractional CO(2) laser for the treatment of atrophic acne scars. J Cosmet Dermatol 2021;20(2):481–90.

56. Hazen PG, Hazen BP. Hidradenitis suppurativa: successful treatment using carbon dioxide laser excision and marsupialization. Dermatol Surg 2010;36(2):208–13.

57. Madan V, Hindle E, Hussain W, et al. Outcomes of treatment of nine cases of recalcitrant severe hidradenitis suppurativa with carbon dioxide laser. Br J Dermatol 2008;159(6):1309–14.

58. Acikel C, Ergun O, Ulkur E, et al. Camouflage of self-inflicted razor blade incision scars with carbon dioxide laser resurfacing and thin skin grafting. Plast Reconstr Surg 2005;116(3):798–804.

59. Du F, Yu Y, Zhou Z, et al. Early treatment using fractional CO2 laser before skin suture during scar revision surgery in Asians. J Cosmet Laser Ther 2018;20(2):102–5.

60. Zhang Y, Liu Y, Cai B, et al. Improvement of Surgical Scars by Early Intervention With Carbon Dioxide Fractional Laser. Lasers Surg Med 2020;52(2):137–48.

Chemical Peels

Richard H. Bensimon, MD

KEYWORDS

- Facial resurfacing • Deep chemical peeling • Croton oil peel • Baker peel • Laser resurfacing
- Lipofilling + croton oil peeling

KEY POINTS

- Facial resurfacing is often overlooked but it is essential for rejuvenation.
- Lasers are inadequate for difficult wrinkles, particularly around the mouth.
- Croton oil peels yield excellent and long-lasting results.
- Misconceptions about the danger and difficulty of croton oil peels.
- Croton oil peels are accessible and feasible for any practitioner.

INTRODUCTION

It is the opinion of this author that the resurfacing of facial skin is an indispensable part of facial rejuvenation and that it has received much less attention. This is regrettable because even the best performed facelift with "old" skin will still look old. Moreover, surgeons understand that surgery has no effect on perioral rhytids and a facelift can make them more noticeable because of the contrast that is created. It should also be noted that aging changes of the skin itself can have greater importance to patients than jowls or loose skin.

Ablative CO_2 lasers are a possibility, but hypopigmentation and a difficult recovery have limited their use. Erbium lasers are an option and in experienced hands are a viable alternative, although deep wrinkles around the mouth and eyes are incompletely treated. Fractionated lasers have proven ineffective for deep wrinkles.

The purpose of this article is to explore deep chemical peels with croton oil and give a practical guideline so that practitioners may consider this terrific technique.

The first easily reproducible formula dates back to 1962 when Thomas Baker published a practical formula consisting of phenol, croton oil, water, and a surgical soap, Septisol, to act as a surfactant. This formula was certainly effective in improving deep wrinkles, but it was troubled by significant hypopigmentation and an unnatural porcelain look. The perceived lack of control in judging depth and the reputation of cardiotoxicity limited the utility of this peel and it did not enjoy wide acceptance.

The crucial step in the development of modern chemical peels came about from the work of Gregory Hetter.[1] Hetter, a plastic surgeon in Las Vegas, frustrated by his options for resurfacing, took a scientific approach in the hope of better understanding the Baker formula. Hetter experimented by performing a number of peels with different combinations of the ingredients and discovered that phenol alone has little effect. Adding croton oil to the phenol at different concentrations resulted in deeper peels proportional to the concentrations of the croton oil. An analysis of the classic Baker formula showed for the first time that the croton oil concentration was very high at 2.1%—responsible for the results as well as the hypopigmentation. Recognizing that croton oil, not phenol, was the peeling agent, Hetter could now alter the concentration so as to give the clinical result without negatively altering the quality of the skin. An important observation was that the lack of control ascribed to phenol was simply that the croton oil concentration was so high that it immediately peeled to the point of hypopigmentation. This may seem a small difference, but it is actually a fundamental change that ushered in the modern era of chemical peeling. Being able to choose the croton oil concentration allowed the procedure to be performed superficially or deep and make it

Plastic Surgery, Bensimon Center, 1200 NW Naito Parkway, Suite 390, Portland, OR 97209, USA
E-mail address: bensi@aol.com

Facial Plast Surg Clin N Am 31 (2023) 475–494
https://doi.org/10.1016/j.fsc.2023.05.006
1064-7406/23/© 2023 Elsevier Inc. All rights reserved.

applicable to all ages and skin types. An important improvement was that different croton oil concentrations could be used in different areas of the face depending on skin thickness and clinical need. A critical change was that with weaker croton oil concentrations, the application technique became an important factor in determining the depth reached. The entire process is slowed down so that the surgeon can observe the skin changes and stop at the depth deemed appropriate. In this manner, the surgeon is in precise control and the process becomes orderly and predictable.[2]

PREOPERATIVE PLANNING

On a basic level, a chemical peel is a controlled chemical burn done in the expectation of creating an anatomic change in the dermis via an increased deposition of collagen and elastin.

As this is a true injury, it is followed by a somewhat peculiar recovery for which the patient must be prepared. It is important to note that any technique, be it peeling or laser, that intends to give a real result has a real recovery period. Any modality that touts an easy recovery will also have little result.

The immediate post-peel phase is not long and typically not uncomfortable, but it is unusual; therefore, the surgeon must be completely honest with the patient. Detailed photographs of the day-by-day recovery are shown to the patient and possibly to a spouse or caregiver. The surgeon must set an upbeat and optimistic although realistic tone. Patients do well if they are well informed and bring a good attitude. The reward is a dramatic and remarkably stable improvement in skin texture which is not possible with any other modality.

The skin is prepared prior to the peel to prevent pigmentary changes such as hyperpigmentation and to have the skin in optimal condition. The main medications are tretinoin and hydroquinone 4%. The effect is to stabilize the epidermis, stimulate the dermis, increase collagen content, increase vascularity, and suppress melanocytes.

The preparation begins 4 to 6 weeks before peeling with tretinoin 0.05% or 0.1% at night and hydroquinone 4% 2 times daily.

The preparation is stopped about 4 days prior to the procedure to allow the epidermis to normalize.

There are differences of opinion whether this skin preparation is necessary, but my experience has been that there is more erythema if avoided. In darker skinned individuals, the preparation is all the more important. In fair-skinned, light-eyed individuals, the bleaching aspect (hydroquinone) can be omitted.

PREPARATION OF THE SOLUTION

The preparation of the acid solution is a critical step that should be performed by the operating surgeon. The ingredients are the same as in the classic Baker peel, namely water, phenol, croton oil, and Septisol. Phenol is a solid crystalline substance that is soluble in water. Standard solutions found in pharmacies and dermatologic suppliers are 88% or 89% phenol. Phenol has a corrosive effect on skin by denaturing the protein and allowing it to pass into the dermis.

Croton oil is a natural oil extracted from the seeds of *Croton tiglium,* a small tree native to India and Southeast Asia. Croton oil is very caustic and will result in a full-thickness ulcer if applied full strength on the skin. When properly diluted and applied, however, croton oil can bring about dramatic results.

Septisol is a surgical soap consisting of liquid hexachlorophene that serves as a surfactant to allow adequate mixing of the aqueous and oil components. Recently, there has been a problem with Septisol in that it has been banned by the FDA due to issues with triclosan, a preservative. This has nothing to do with its use in peeling, but the end result is that it is no longer available.

Young Pharmaceuticals (youngpharm.com, Wetherfield, CT) has formulated an excellent substitute called Novisol. This is also a surfactant, but its action is different, and it results in a stable solution that lasts 45 minutes. Novisol is used in the same volume as Septisol. Because of the stability of the solution, it may appear that the action using Novisol may be a little weaker. The only repercussion of this is that the highest concentration used may be 1.2% rather than 0.8% on deeper wrinkles such as around the mouth (see below). The water used is regular tap water.

The ingredients are arranged in glass bowls in the order they will be added. Various sized syringes are available along with a glass or metal funnel and sterile gloves for protection. Once readied, the acids can be stored in opaque glass containers and sealed with phenolic cone-lined, leak-proof caps (SKS-bottle.com, bottlesandmore.com). These solutions are stable for an extended period of time.

Original formulas involved using drops of croton oil. The problem with this is that the volume of a drop is not uniform leading to variability and a drop cannot be subdivided, limiting the options. A very practical solution provided by Hetter was to prepare a standard phenol/croton oil solution using larger volumes that would be then further diluted with the other ingredients. The standard or "stock solution" is made by mixing 24 mL of 88% or 89% phenol with 1 mL of croton oil. By using larger volumes of the ingredients, they are easily measured with accuracy using standard syringes and a multitude of concentrations are possible.[3]

Standard tables are available showing the specific volumes of each ingredient to arrive at the final croton oil concentration. The final phenol concentration in these formulas is 35% (**Table 1**).

An examination of the standard formulas shows that the volumes of water and Novisol remain constant at 5.5 mL and 0.5 mL, respectively. The values that change are the relative volumes of phenol and stock solution (which contains phenol and croton oil). The sum of the volumes of the 88% phenol and stock solution is 4 mL in each of the formulas.

It is very important to remember that the croton oil concentration of stock solution is very high at 4% and should never be applied directly on the skin without further dilution. For a reference, the Baker formula had a croton oil concentration of 2.1%.

To make weaker concentrations, one first mixes 0.4% or 0.2% solutions and these are further diluted using the formulas in the table. The final volume is 4 mL, and the final phenol concentration remains at 35%. This formula is very useful because whatever starting concentration is used will be diluted by one-fourth, that is, 1 mL of X% croton oil solution + 1.2 mL phenol + 1.8 mL water will yield $\frac{1}{4}$ X% solution.

Since Hetter's publications in 2000, 35% phenol concentration has become standard, but useful variations are possible. For example, there are darker skinned individuals who may have less wrinkling and more pigmentary issues. In this instance, a low croton oil concentration formula is chosen and then the relative volume of water and phenol are changed to elevate the phenol concentration to 50% or 60%. For example, to change the phenol concentration to 60% in the 0.1% croton oil, 4 mL formula, the total volume of phenol needed (X) is determined by x/4 mL = .6; than X = 2.4 mL. The 1 mL of 0.4% croton oil solution brings 0.35 mL phenol (35% phenol solution), this leaves 2.05 mL of phenol lacking. 0.88X = 2.05 mL represents the volume of 88% phenol needed, or 2.33 mL. In the formula, the volume of phenol and the volume of water add up to 3 mL; substituting 2.33 mL of phenol and 0.67 mL of water in the formula results in a 60% phenol solution. Understanding and manipulating the formulas results in enormous variability.

INTRAOPERATIVE ROUTINE

Traditionally, deep chemical peels have been performed under general anesthesia or intravenous sedation due to the intense discomfort of the chemical burn. Following induction, standard sensory blocks are performed with bupivacaine with epinephrine and ketorolac tromethamine 30 to 60 mg is administered as an adjunct to anesthesia.

This is a viable approach which I have used for years and is certainly acceptable. There have been recent developments that have led to an alternative technique. Experience treating pigmented spots on my hand with 50% or 60% phenol demonstrated to me that there is an initial period of stinging lasting 10 to 15 seconds after which the skin is very anesthetic, even when slowly twirling a needle to the point of bleeding. This is explained by phenol causing a neurolytic effect that reversibly prevents the transmission of nerve impulses.

This phenol effect is potentially useful; I began peeling by first applying a pass of 50% or 60% phenol. This was initially stimulating, but it quickly subsided, and the peel could proceed. This technique may do away with the need for sensory blocks, but further experience is needed. My observation has been that this use of phenol leads to a relatively pain free emergence and a comfortable post-peel course.[4] The anesthetic use of phenol is very useful in awake segmental peels. To make 50% phenol, one simply dilutes 10 mL of 88% phenol with 7.5 mL water.

Ophthalmic ointment and corneal protection are not used because phenol can dissolve in the ointment or become trapped under a protector

Table 1 Croton oil peel formulas using 35% phenol vehicle				
Croton Oil %	0.2%	0.4%	0.8%	1.2%
Water	5.5 mL.	5.5 mL.	5.5 mL.	5.5 mL.
Novisol	0.5 mL.	0.5 mL.	0.5 mL.	0.5 mL.
USP phenol 88%	3.5 mL.	3.0 mL.	2.0 mL.	1.0 mL.
Stock solution Containing phenol and croton oil	0.5 mL.	1.0 mL.	2.0 mL.	3.0 mL.
Total	10 mL.	10 mL.	10 mL.	10 mL.

0.1% = 1 mL of 0.4% + 1.2 mL phenol+ 1.8 mL. water.
0.05% = 1 mL of 0.2% + 1.2 mL phenol + 1.8 mL water.
1/4X% = 1 mL of X% + 1.2 mL phenol + 1.8 mL water.
Stock solution = 24 mL phenol + 1 mL croton oil.
(0.04 mL croton oil) or 4% croton oil.
(1 mL stock solution).
50% Phenol = 10mL. Phenol + 7mL. Water + 0.5 mL. Novisol
Warning: The Stock Solution is only meant to be diluted and should never be applied on the skin full strength.

preventing complete flushing out if it becomes necessary. Constant vigilance around the eyes is essential.

The fear of cardiac toxicity due to phenol requires careful consideration. It had been the belief that peels performed under general anesthesia but without blocks led to intense stimulation due to the high concentration of croton oil and this led to the cardiac irritability. The general belief was that with proper local blocks and performing a full-face peel is no less than 45 minutes, there was a little danger.

A recent experience during a live surgery course was very elucidating: An overzealous novice applied peeling solution over a large portion of the face much too quickly and a multitude of worrisome arrhythmias were seen. The decision was to back off, actively hydrate and do nothing. In 10 minutes, the electrocardiogram reverted to normal and remained so.

This important episode has led me to conclude that (1) phenol is absorbed and can lead to significant arrhythmias and (2) this is an orderly and predictable process that is related to speed of application. If the peel is not hurried and a full-face peel takes 45 minutes to 1 hour, there is no fear of cardiac irritability. A screening electrocardiogram (EKG) is performed in patients aged over 65 years or if there is a history of arrhythmias.

The first step is to degrease the skin to allow even absorption of the solutions. Ask the patient not to apply anything on the skin on the morning of the peel. Acetone is the best agent for degreasing.

The environment must be quiet and organized, not hectic and hurried. This is especially true around the eyes: Corneal protection and ophthalmic ointments are not used, and extreme care is the sole protection. The head of the bed is elevated to prevent the solution from rolling into the eyes. The applying instrument, be it a sponge or cotton tipped applicator, should never be so wet that it can drip. Never crossing over the eyes with the applying hand is extremely important and should become second nature, not unlike sterile technique. The surgeon's hand must be dry so as not to apply acid where it is not wanted. The best way to insure this is to clip a surgical towel to the surgeon's scrub shirt shoulder and draped over the front, always at the ready for wiping the hands.

The bottle containing the solution is shaken to evenly mix the ingredients. A small volume of the desired solution is poured into a small glass bowl, and a second bowl is placed over it to prevent escape of the vapors. A small fan held by an assistant helps dissipate these vapors, and the now ubiquitous N-95 masks are useful. A calm, measured demeanor by the surgeon completes the picture.

The most common applying material is a 2-inch by 2-inch gauze, preferably synthetic fiber, which is less abrasive. Cotton-tipped applicators are useful for the eyelids and to target individual wrinkles. The splintered wooden end of the applicator or toothpicks are also useful. The gauze is folded twice to decrease the size and be more precise. It is now dipped in the solution and wrung out so that it is moist and not so wet that it could drip. The gauze is set down in a safe place, and the hands are dried with the clipped towel to prevent inadvertent application of the acid where it is not wanted. This is particularly important in segmental peels where the error would be obvious. The applying hand should never cross over the eyes.

Once the gauze is applied to the skin, the effect is seen in 10 to 15 seconds depending on how wet the gauze is and the concentration of the croton oil solution. The action of the acid is to coagulate and precipitate the protein of the skin forming a "frost", which is varying degrees of a white appearance. As more passes are made, the depth of the skin reached is assessed by the degree and quality of the white appearance. With increased depth, the frost becomes progressively more dense, solid, and opaque. On a cellular level, this represents the coagulating action of the acid passing through the epidermis to the papillary dermis (juncture between epidermis and dermis). As the peel passes from the papillary dermis to the upper and mid-reticular dermis, the frosting becomes a dull, flat white. Unlike trichloroacetic acid (TCA) peels, the action is quick and there is no need to wait a few minutes to see the final effect. Unlike some other peels, this change is irreversible. The only control available to the surgeon is that if the application is too wet, quickly blotting it will diminish the action.

FACTORS DETERMINING THE DEPTH OF THE PEEL

Older peels with a croton oil concentration of 2.1% were problematic because they immediately peeled to a depth resulting in hypopigmentation—there was no control. A key concept of modern peels is that with lower croton oil concentrations, the entire process is slowed down and there is ample opportunity to gauge the depth of peel. In this manner, the application technique, which is wholly under the control of the surgeon, becomes the determining factor of the depth reached. The number of coats applied has a cumulative effect and with a particular concentration, a damp sponge can be rubbed multiple times, variable pressure can be used, or the gauze can be wetter and fewer passes made. The same depth can be reached using different techniques or different concentrations. By the same token, a weak concentration can be repeatedly applied and lead to deep involvement.

JUDGING THE DEPTH OF THE PEEL

The key to a successful resurfacing is choosing and safely reaching the appropriate endpoint. A superficial peel wounds the epidermis, and although it can improve pigmentation and give a bright look, it does not improve real wrinkles. A medium–depth peel reaches the papillary dermis. Deep peels go to the upper and mid-reticular dermis, and it is this layer that must be reached to have significant improvement of stubborn wrinkles. The recovery depends on the depth reached and croton oil peels require more time for reepithelialization and resolution. Any other modality touting a quicker recovery, such as fractionated laser, will not have a similar result. Typically, in most cases, different depths are reached in different areas of the face depending on skin thickness and clinical need. Peeling deeper than the mid-reticular dermis can lead to hypopigmentation and scarring.

During the peel, specific attention must be paid to the appearance and quality of the frost as this is the way to judge the depth. The clues to look for are background color, "thickness" and opacity. A thin, transparent frost with a pinkish background means that acid has traversed through the epidermis into the papillary dermis. There is a quality of translucence that allows visualization of the horizontal vessels of the dermis resulting in the pink color (**Fig. 1**). This may well be the endpoint in some areas. With further application, the acid passes into the reticular dermis and forms a solid, opaque, evenly colored organized frost (**Fig. 2**). The action of the acid has destroyed the more superficial dermal vessels and the opacity does not allow visualization of the deeper subdermal plexus; therefore, the pink background is not seen. In thicker areas, such as around the mouth, the peel is stopped at this point and the frost is allowed to subside, or "defrost." If the upper to mid-reticular dermis has been successfully reached, the defrosting takes about 15 minutes, and the skin takes on a reddish–brown overtone (**Fig. 3**). This a very reliable sign and if it is not seen, further peeling may be needed. A gray–white appearance of the frost suggests reaching the lower reticular dermis and is not recommended.

Another visual cue to assess the depth of peel, especially in thin skin like the eyelids, is epidermal sliding. Epidermal sliding is a phenomenon that occurs when the peel reaches the papillary dermis and the tight bond between the epidermis and dermis is broken, allowing the epidermis to slide as a single sheet. This sliding disappears when the peel goes deeper and the epidermis and dermis bond as a single protein block.

The progression from superficial to deep is gradual, orderly, and the visual changes are easily recognizable and predictable. The advantage of modern peels is that the surgeon has control. This is based on going slow enough to recognize the various stages, stop at the appropriate depth and go no deeper.

Full-face Peel

The following is a step-by-step description of my approach to a full-face peel. The patient is sedated and has received clonidine 0.1 mg p.o. prior. This is based on empirical experience that it helps prevent arrhythmias. Endotracheal gas anesthesia is an option, but it is my preference to avoid it. The head of the bed is slightly elevated to prevent drops from flowing into the eyes. The skin is degreased with acetone, and no ophthalmic ointment or corneal protection is used. Sterile surgical gloves offer more protection than nonsterile ones. A surgical towel is clipped to the shoulder of the scrub shirt and draped over the front.

The various solutions have been pre-mixed and placed in clearly labeled bottles. Small glass bowls are available to pour solution into for dipping. Extra gauze and irrigating ophthalmic solution are kept within easy reach in case washing out of the eyes should be needed. The bottle of the solution to be used is gently shaken to evenly mix the ingredients and a small amount is poured into a glass bowl. A 2 × 2 gauze is folded twice, dipped into the bowl, and then wrung out until damp but not dripping. A second glass bowl is placed over the first to trap the fumes. The damp gauze is set in a safe place, the hands are wiped on the clipped towel, and then the gauze is retrieved for peeling.

I start on the perioral area as I usually want to peel to the reticular dermis and then move on to other areas as the mouth defrosts. Starting on the upper lips, a first pass is made, and the skin is examined. I usually use 0.8% concentration or possibly 1.2% with the solutions using Novisol on deeper wrinkles. A light frost appears and as more passes are made, the frost becomes denser and more concentrated. A translucent frost with a pink background means that the papillary dermis has been reached. With more passes, redipping

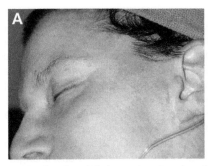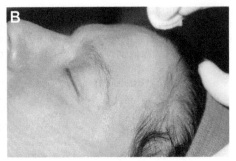

Fig. 1. Progressive frosting. (*A*) The patient is sedated and the skin degreased. (*B*) The first passes are made, and a thin translucent frost appears with a pink background.

the gauze as necessary, the frost becomes progressively more dense, more opaque, losing the pink background as the upper reticular dermis is reached. As previously mentioned, this is a slow, orderly process and the surgeon can stop at any point if a lesser peel is desired.

The skin is stretched to allow even application of the acid between wrinkles. The commissures are also spread and respond well to deep peeling. The lower lips and chin area are peeled in a similar manner to an opaque solid white frost. The margin of the peel is the inferior border of the mandible and chin (**Fig. 4**). The peel can now proceed to the next area while monitoring the defrosting over the next 15 to 20 minutes, observing for the tan, red-brown overtones. This confirms having reached the upper to mid-reticular dermis. If this color change is not evident or too faint, the area can be repealed. The next area is the glabella and nose, which have roughly similar thickness as the mouth; the glabella in particular can have deeply etched lines and can be peeled to the reticular dermis. The lower nose does not wrinkle, but "roughness" and deep pores respond well to similarly deep peeling.

The skin of the forehead is thicker centrally and thins out superiorly and laterally. Aside from the

glabella and transverse lines, the forehead does not have generalized wrinkles. A common approach is to peel centrally with 0.4%, feathering superiorly. The rest of the forehead is peeled with 0.2% to the papillary dermis and peeling lightly in the temporal area as it is delicate and not usually wrinkled (**Fig. 5**). The transverse lines and glabella lines can be targeted deeper, as will be discussed later. The peels do not affect hair growth so peeling should continue to hairline and brows to avoid a demarcation. Treating the dynamic lines of the upper face with botulinum toxin 2 weeks prior is recommended to decrease mobility during healing.

The face between the eyes and mouth are peeled next. The skin of the posterior face is densely attached and less mobile, therefore usually less wrinkled. The posterior area is usually peeled with 0.2% to the papillary dermis, with light application in the preauricular area which is delicate (**Fig. 6**). Peeling should continue to the sideburn, tragus, and earlobe. The earlobe responds nicely and can be peeled with 0.4%.

The anterior face, showing more mobility, is usually more wrinkled. Depending on the individual case, this area is peeled with 0.2% or 0.4% to the papillary dermis or slightly deeper and

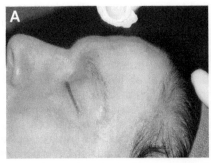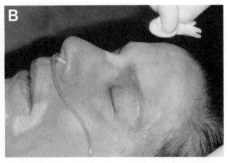

Fig. 2. Progressive frosting. (*A*) As more passes area made, the frost becomes more organized and opaque, with a pink background still evident. This denotes reaching the papillary dermis. (*B*) After more passes in the thicker glabella, the frost has become thicker, organized, and opaque. The peel has passed into the reticular dermis.

The eyelids are an excellent area for peeling, especially the lower eyelids, because they can show great improvement and are very predictable. The skin is very thin, but it responds well to a weak solution such as 0.1%. The solution is applied with 2 cotton-tipped applicators that are dipped into the bottle after it has been shaken. The wet applicators are touched to a gauze or drape to slightly dry them, and then applied to the skin. The peel begins in the lower part of the lid and then proceeds gradually superiorly approximating the ciliary margin. The relative dampness of the applicators and the number of passes made determine the depth. The cheek is gently pulled down to fully expose the skin and smooth out the wrinkles. With progressive passes, the friction of the application will demonstrate epidermal sliding and the frost will become an even white color. When the cheek is released, the soft tissue moves up and the degree of epidermal sliding can be easily seen. When the epidermis is loose and there is an even white frost, the opposite lid can be addressed. After defrosting, a prominent wrinkle or redundancy may be seen at mid-height that can be repealed, possibly with 0.05% solution (**Fig. 7**). Having a detailed photograph present is useful to see the precise location of the wrinkles.

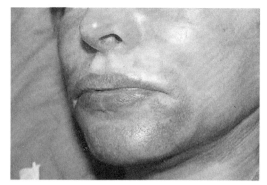

Fig. 3. The red-brown appearance after defrosting is a reliable sign that the reticular dermis has been reached.

individual wrinkles can be targeted as necessary. The anterior face can be tricky, because on occasion, there can be deep wrinkles in an area where the skin is not as thick; therefore, the patient must be advised that complete correction may not be possible. The peel should extend to about 1 cm below the mandible and the entire corridor of the mandibular border between the mandibular angle and the geniomandibular groove is delicate and rarely wrinkled; therefore, it should be peeled lightly.

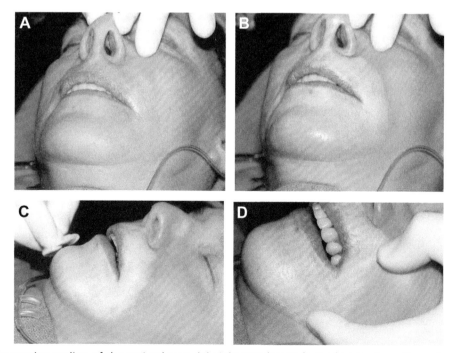

Fig. 4. Progressive peeling of the perioral area. (*A*) Light translucent frost of upper lip as the early passes are made. (*B*) More passes have been made in the upper lip and the frost is solid and opaque. The lower lip and chin still show a pink background. (*C*) Both upper and lower lips/chin demonstrate solid, dense frost indicative of reaching the reticular dermis. (*D*) The commisures do well and can be specifically targeted.

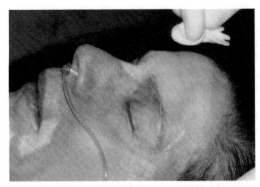

Fig. 5. The peel of the forehead is deeper centrally, tapering superiorly and laterally. The glabella is often peeled to the reticular dermis, whereas the superior and lateral skin shows a light frost with a pink background, which represents peeling to the papillary dermis.

Because of the tightness that is created, precipitating an ectropion is always a possibility, so testing the laxity of the lid preoperatively is important. If there is concern about laxity, a preemptive canthopexy or tarsorrhaphy suture can be performed or sequential lighter peels can be done. Patients may experience tightness in the lower lids after peeling, but this responds promptly to upward massage.

The skin of the upper lids responds to peeling by shrinking, which looks quite nice and can mimic a blepharoplasty. If laxity is present, peel with 0.1% and it is usually stopped at the tarsal fold. If there is laxity below the fold, the peel can approximate the lashes. One nuisance of peeling the upper lid is that the eye may swell shut, usually until the next day.

The peel is then extended onto the neck with a very dilute solution of 0.25% or even weaker. This is done with very light, wispy strokes and a barely moist sponge leaving a faint frost that is

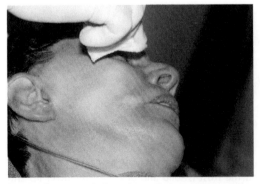

Fig. 6. The central face is peeled to the papillary dermis. Deeper wrinkles can be individually targeted.

scattered and disorganized. This peel is done only to prevent a line of demarcation and not to improve wrinkles; the neck skin is delicate and lacks the healing potential of the face. Attempting to improve wrinkles is likely to cause hypopigmentation or scarring. A weak TCA peel in the neck is an option and liposuction of the neck with any peeling is not recommended. Likewise, a brow lift, even if performed at a deep level, is to be avoided.

At this point, the entire face is inspected to see if any further peeling is needed. Areas where the intention was to reach the mid-reticular dermis are examined for the red-brown color. If not present or faint, they should be repealed. If there is uneven blending of areas peeled with different concentrations, then a light overpeel with a dilute solution such as 0.1% is needed. This is most common in the midface.

Precise peeling of individual deeper rhytids without affecting the surrounding areas is an extremely valuable tool, especially in the perioral area, chin, glabella, and forehead. A wetter cotton-tipped applicator is used to paint the individual line and then quickly drying it as the frost appears. This is repeated until the desired depth is reached (**Fig. 8**). This is particularly useful in stubborn radial lines around the mouth and can have a profound effect. Transverse forehead lines are stubborn, but improvement can be expected from this technique. This is also true for glabella lines, transverse nasal lines, and crow's feet.

Various croton oil concentrations have been recommended in the previous sections, but keep in mind that the concentration of the solution is only one variable, and the surgeon needs to monitor the appearance of the frost at all times and decide the depth at which to stop. Repeated passes of whatever concentration will have additive effect and the safety of a weaker concentration is a relative one.

The patient should be well hydrated and under cardiac monitoring during a full-face peel. The surgeon should be aware of the pulse rate, and if it increases, back off until it slows down. Resist the temptation of peeling too fast, especially as experience is gained. A full-face peel should take between 45 minutes and 1 hour. If arrhythmias are seen, stop the peel for some minutes until the rhythm reverts to normal. In all likelihood, treatment will not be necessary.

Aftercare

Dealing with the skin after the peel is perhaps the most challenging aspect of deep chemical peels. There is, in essence, an open wound and the aim

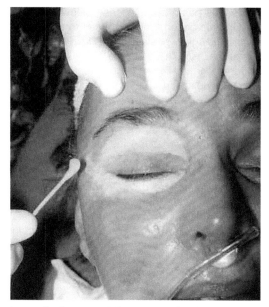

Fig. 7. The lower eyelids are peeled with 0.1% croton oil solution to a point of epidermal sliding and an even white frost. The upper lids are peeled with 0.1% solution or possibly 0.05%, depending on the degree of laxity. The peel stops at the tarsal fold unless obvious laxity is seen below the fold.

is to provide a good environment to promote reepithelialization in the fastest time with the least difficulty for the patient. Keep in mind that to obtain a significant result, there must be an injury into the

dermis, and as a result, there is a real recovery. Any other process that has a quick recovery has not adequately injured the dermis and will not give a comparable result.

The traditional technique of after care, which I used for the first 14 years of my peeling experience, involved using triple antibiotic ointment mixed with lidocaine jelly and constantly applying it to the face. This technique works and is a viable option, but it is messy and gives the patient a dramatic view of the "aftermath" and requires constant touching of the face. Moreover, sensitization to the antibiotics can cause breakouts and rashes. Milia were common, and there was the impression that the subsequent erythema was more intense.

The following is my present regimen which I instituted to improve the patient experience and have used successfully for the last 8 years. Once the peel is finished and all the frosting has subsided, all the peeled areas are covered with zinc oxide tape. This is the pink tape commonly used by anesthesia providers to secure the endotracheal tube. Petrolatum ointment is applied to the brow and hairline to prevent sticking, and no taping is done to the skin of the upper lid below the tarsal fold (**Fig. 9**).

Typically, when patients awaken from the peel, they may feel some stinging which is not intense and may or may not necessitate medication. This is not long lasting, and when discharged in about

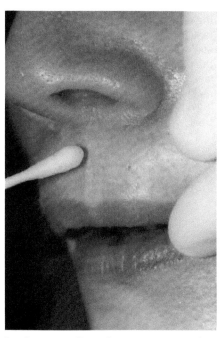
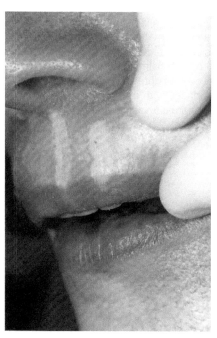

Fig. 8. Precise deeper peeling of more pronounced wrinkles is possible with a wetter application, then quickly drying as the frost appears. This is repeated until the desired depth is reached. This is an extremely valuable tool in the perioral area.

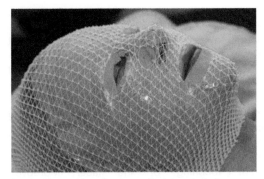

Fig. 9. Zinc-oxide take is applied to peeled areas at the end of the peel.

1 hour, they are comfortable. Unlike the very difficult recovery from the Baker peel (and ablative lasers), this is usually the last discomfort felt.

The tape mask remains in place overnight, at which point the patient returns to the office. The tape mask is removed from inferior to superior without difficulty and without discomfort. The patient should be warned that any discomfort felt is simply some hair caught in the tape. An inconvenience of peeling the upper lid is that it may swell shut the night of the peel or the tape may impede the lid from opening. Vision is restored the next day when the tape is removed (**Fig. 10**).

The peeled skin is examined and gently cleansed with a saline gauze in order to remove any loose fibrous material. The edge of a tongue depressor can also be used to gently "shave" the skin.

The next step is to mix bismuth subgallate powder with water to create an even, creamy paste with a consistency reminiscent of cake frosting. A small bit of ophthalmic gel can be added to give a more even texture. The paste is applied to all peeled surfaces with a tongue depressor or a mini silicone spatula (available in a kitchen store). A fan-shaped makeup brush works well on the eyelids. The paste is not applied below the tarsal fold. Organic coconut oil is applied to the vermillion and the lightly peeled neck (**Fig. 11**).

Once the bismuth mask is on, it is allowed to dry and form a crust. The patient is admonished that from this point on, they are to strictly avoid touching the face. Over the next 7 to 12 days, the skin beneath will reepithelialize and shed the crust piecemeal. Again, the patient is advised not to pick at, wash, or touch the face. At about day 7, the patient is seen and a heavy petroleum ointment is applied to any remaining crust and allowed to seep in during that day. On day 8, the patient can shower gently (deflect the full force of the shower with a hand), gently pat dry with clean hands and clean towel, and re-apply the ointment (which is supplied to the patient) on remaining crust. This is repeated daily until the mask is completely shed and the new pink skin is evident (usually 9–12 days) (**Figs. 12** and **13**).

This approach with the bismuth has the disadvantage of looking bizarre but the typical reaction has been one of amusement and patients are very tolerant of it. The hands-off approach is appreciated, and office visits and worried calls have been significantly cut down in the first 2 weeks. Any questions are easily handled via smartphone photos. The bismuth has proven less reactive than ointment and the post peel erythema is much less.

Once skin is exposed, a medical quality moisturizer is applied with clean hands and continued for the ensuing weeks. Strict sun avoidance is important for the early periods, and usually a physical sun block can be used on the third week giving the patient increased freedom. The erythema can last 8 to 12 weeks but is easily covered with makeup or tinted sunblock.

To be sure, there are many other techniques to treat resurfaced skin, but the tape-bismuth

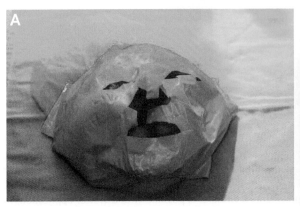
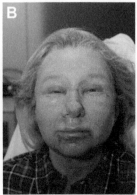

Fig. 10. (*A*) The tape mask is removed the day after the peel. (*B*) Appearance immediately after tape mask removal.

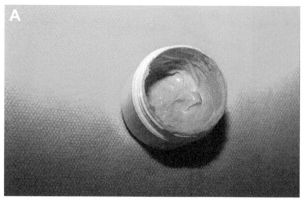
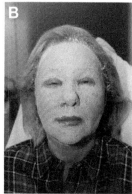

Fig. 11. (*A*) Bismuth subgallate paste. (*B*) Bismuth paste applied to face.

approach has proven to be effective and practical. Some patients may consider the process too onerous, but in reality, the 2-week early recovery is quite short when considering there is no other treatment equal in quality and longevity. As more practitioners perform these peels, an improved aftercare technique may come to light.

Variation of peels

Partial or segmental peels are a possibility but must be done judiciously so as not to create a mismatch in color. This is particularly true in patients with widespread solar damage, making a full-face peel a better choice. For example, if an isolated peel is performed, the true color of the skin will be brought out and this could be in harsh contrast to surrounding sun-damaged skin. In these situations, a lesser peel may be preferable to avoid the need for makeup. Some individuals with isolated upper lip lines without extensive

sun damage elsewhere can benefit from a peel of the mustache area (**Fig. 14**).

The eyelids are an excellent area for segmental peeling. Signs of early aging are often seen first around the eyelids in late 30s to mid-40s. The upper lids exhibit slight redundancy, and the lower lids show crisscrossing, visible wrinkling, and crepiness. These changes are bothersome to patients as they are often the only signs of aging and the myriad of cream and treatments available do little. A simple peel, often performed in the office without anesthesia in 10 minutes, can greatly improve the problem. The thin lid skin, if peeled within the boundary of the orbital rim, responds very well and is easy to hide with makeup or glasses. If more improvement is desired, the peel can be repeated with little expenditure in time or materials. In a real sense, the patient can obtain as smooth a lid as they wish.

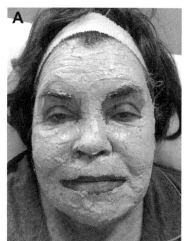
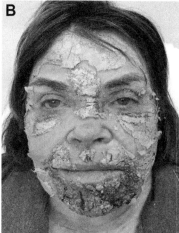
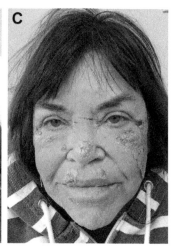

Fig. 12. Process of healing with bismuth subgallate paste. (*A*) Day 1. (*B*) Day 5. (*C*) Day 7. Note that erythema is more where peel is deeper (glabella), but overall is mild.

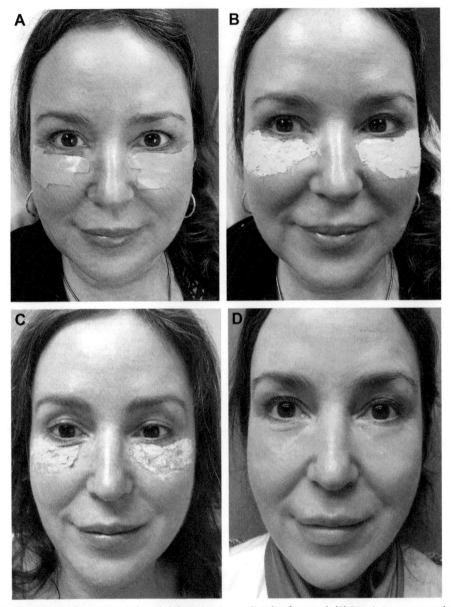

Fig. 13. Healing process for segmental peel. (*A*) Taping immediately after peel. (*B*) Day 1, tape removal and application of bismuth subgallate paste. (*C*) Interim healing. Partial shedding of crust. (*D*) Appearance after complete shedding of crust. Note that erythema is mild and easily concealable.

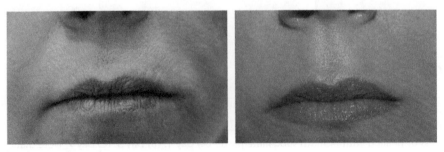

Fig. 14. Isolated mustache peel.

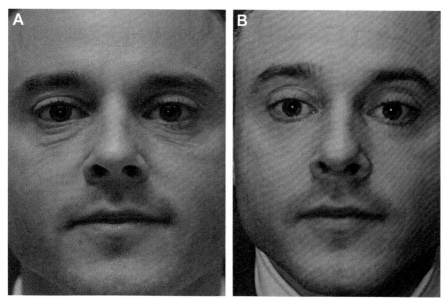

Fig. 15. (*A*) A 44 year old man with crepiness and slight redundancy of lower lid skin as the main expression of aging. A lower lid blepharoplasty might have further accentuated the rounding of his outer canthi. (*B*) Result 6 months after peel of lower eyelids. This is an excellent option for this problem.

There is great versatility in these eyelid peels: If a quicker recovery is needed, a lighter peel can be done with the thought of repeating it at a later time. A lower eyelid peel tightens the anterior lamella and tends to soften the early bulging of fat in younger patients. Likewise, the skin of the upper lid reacts by shrinking, giving a bright, natural look without surgery. The combination of a transconjunctival blepharoplasty and a lower lid peel is an excellent choice that gives predictably good results without changing the shape of the eye (**Figs. 15** and **16**).

An evolving tactic is to peel the eyelids of young patients when this is the only sign of aging. After

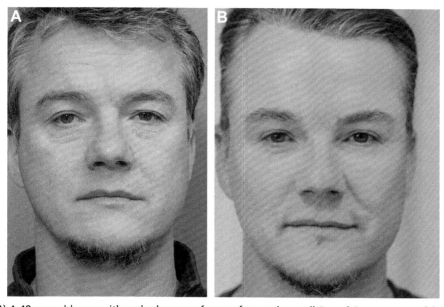

Fig. 16. (*A*) A 48 year old man with early changes of upper face and overall "rough" appearance. (*B*) Result after upper blepharoplasty, neuromodulators, skin care, and lower lid peel. Relatively simple procedures have produced considerable impact.

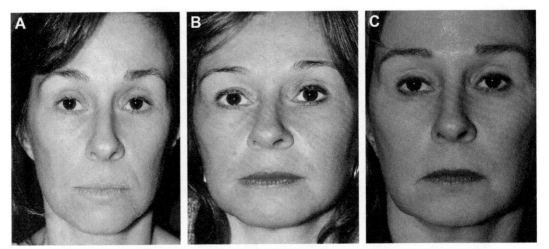

Fig. 17. (*A*) A 45 year old woman with generalized elastosis and chin wrinkles. (*B*) One year post-peel. The skin looks healthier with bright reflection of light and improvement of chin wrinkles. (*C*) Six years postoperatively. There is remarkable stability of results.

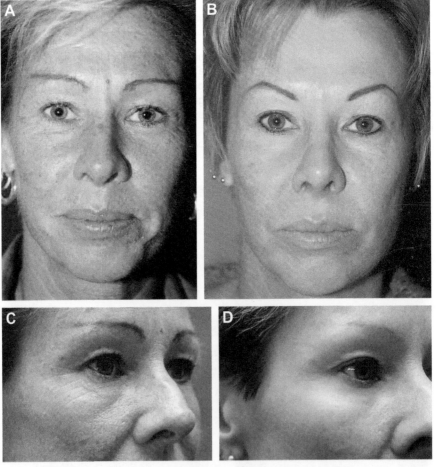

Fig. 18. (*A, C*) A 47 year old woman with widespread sun damage, elastosis, pigmentary changes, and opaque skin (*B*) 4 years after croton oil peel. Global improvement in the quality of the skin and even pigmentation area evident. (*D*) Detail of periorbital area 1 year after peeling. The qualitative improvement consists of softening of the hard lizard-like skin and the natural absorption and reflection of light.

some years go by and there is some further deterioration, the peel is repeated, and the skin is brought back to its previous condition. This is an effective way to keep up with aging. These peels (and any touchups) can be done with mild oral sedation and a first pass of 50% phenol. After about 12 seconds of stinging, the skin is numb, and you can proceed to the next lid. Once all areas are anesthetic, the peel can proceed.

This preemptive approach can be applied to the whole face as fine wrinkling and the dullness of solar elastosis begins to appear. This may be the situation in younger patients not contemplating any surgery, but also not seeing adequate results from superficial peels, microdermabrasion, etc. In these circumstances, a lighter peel can be done, targeting any problem areas such as the eyelids or lip lines. The recovery will be quicker, but the result will be more profound than with TCA or fractionated laser. Any persistent wrinkle can be easily touched up. This treatment plan is applicable to a large portion of the population, and if repeated appropriately, will prevent more obvious aging.

Results

In its basics, croton oil peels injure the skin to a particular level and elicit an acute inflammatory response that stimulates the deposition of collagen and elastin. Histology of peeled skin shows a significant new layer of collagen in the dermis that is aligned in an orderly way and is remarkably stable for years, even decades. The positive result in a patient in their 60s can be considered permanent. The qualitative improvement of the skin is by means of a true regenerative process that changes the skin anatomy. The skin looks younger because, in a real sense, younger skin has been created. The haphazard arrangement of epidermal cells is reordered: Light

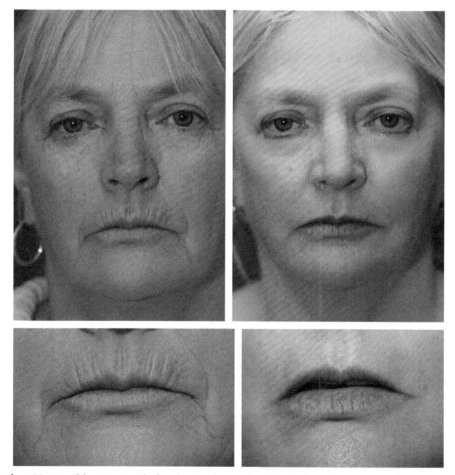

Fig. 19. Left, a 59 year old woman with the classic ashen, sallow look of sun damage, prominent upper lip lines, and rough chin skin. Right, 1 year after croton oil peeling. Generalized improvement of skin quality and pigment, along with stark improvement of upper lip lines and elevation of the vermillion. No other modality has equaled these results.

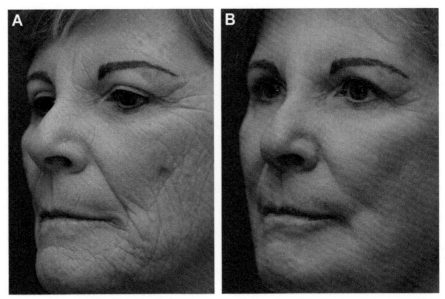

Fig. 20. (*A*) A facelift on this 65 year old woman without resurfacing would be an aesthetic failure as the prominent lines of the face would be minimally improved and around the mouth and upper face, not at all (*B*) 1 year after croton oil peeling. It could be argued that the peel has provided more global rejuvenation than surgery.

penetrates the dermis and is reflected back brightly, replacing the dull, ashen, sallow look of sun damage and elastosis. The generalized qualitative improvement of the skin radiates the luminescence of youth. There is an intangible quality that no surgery can provide. In fact, the results of a well-done facelift without radiant skin are incomplete and still look old. The longevity of peels is unequaled by any other process and rather than showing loss of effect, the skin appears to improve with time. **Figs. 17–23** are representative of the results that can be seen with these deep chemical peels.

Microscopic studies of peeled skin show destruction of actinic keratoses and cancer cells within the dermis before they become clinically

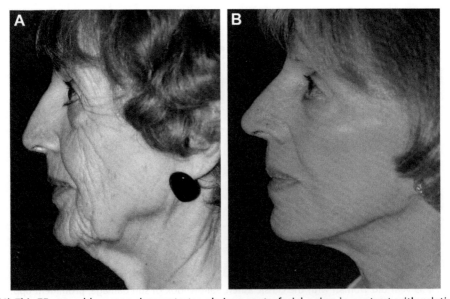

Fig. 21. (*A*) This 75 year old woman demonstrates obvious centrofacial aging in contrast with relatively unaffected posterior face. (*B*) Results 5 years after facelift and 1 year after croton oil peeling. This demonstrates the power of surgery and subsequent peeling (or vice versa).

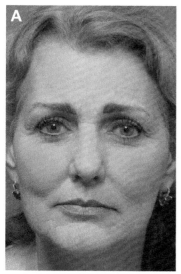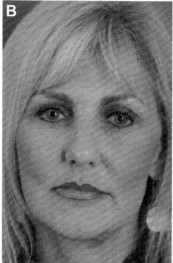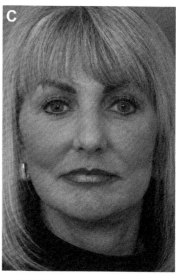

Fig. 22. (*A*) A 63 year old woman with structural changes of aging, jowling, neck laxity, mild hollowing of upper lids, and prominent line especially periorally and upper face. (*B*) One year after facelift and lipofilling. The lack of improvement in the texture distracts from the result and despite the improvements, she still looks "old". (*C*) One and a half years after peeling. A natural, comprehensive result as all 3 components of facial aging (structure, volume, texture) have been addressed.

evident.[5,6] This is to be expected because deep peels go to the depth that these cells are found. The impression of experienced peelers is patients that have been peeled do not develop facial basal cell or squamous cell cancer. Individuals with a previous history of skin cancer show a significant decrease in frequency or even complete eradication. In fact, dermatologic studies have shown that resurfacing techniques are successful in keeping susceptible patients free of non-melanoma skin cancer for the studied 5 years.[7]

In recent years, there has been increased attention in addressing the loss of volume that is seen in aging. The use of fat transfer or lipofilling is becoming more important not only for replenishing lost volume in the face, but also for the regenerative effect of stem cells and epidermal growth factors. With experience, it has been found that lipofilling and croton oil peels can be done at the same time and are very synergistic (**Fig. 24**). This is a powerful combination, and there are many instances where this approach may afford a greater aesthetic impact than a facelift. Of course, if all 3 components of aging are corrected, the result can be very dramatic.

COMPLICATIONS

The main complications of croton oil peels are similar to other deep resurfacing procedures. The most feared complication, scarring, has occurred mainly if the patient picked at their face during the healing process or if they inadvertently transferred genital herpes to the face. This infection is more virulent and has resulted in scarring.

If healing is delayed longer than 14 days or thickening develops, this is suggestive that the peel has reached the deep reticular dermis and scarring may ensue. The suggested treatment is to apply a fluorinated topical steroid 5 days on and 5 days off with careful monitoring. If a scar develops, a useful treatment is the intralesional injection of 5-fluorouracial (5-FU). 5-FU is a common intravenous chemotherapeutic agent with a long history of use by dermatologist and plastic surgeons (**Fig. 25**). The intralesional injection is considered off-label. The schedule of injection can be as frequent as every 1 or 2 weeks, depending on results. Steroid can be mixed with 5-FU, but it appears that 5-FU alone is more effective without the complications of the steroid.

Particular attention should be paid to the temporal area, preauricular area, the geniomandibular border, and the medial upper lid as these areas are delicate and could lead to scarring. The region of the mandibular border from angle to chin should not be overpeeled as it is delicate and rarely wrinkled.

Hypopigmentation can result if the peel goes too deep and was the norm with older peels. This is largely preventable with the modern iteration of these peels as proposed in this article. If an individual has very deep wrinkles and tough leathery skin, it may be necessary to peel so deep as to

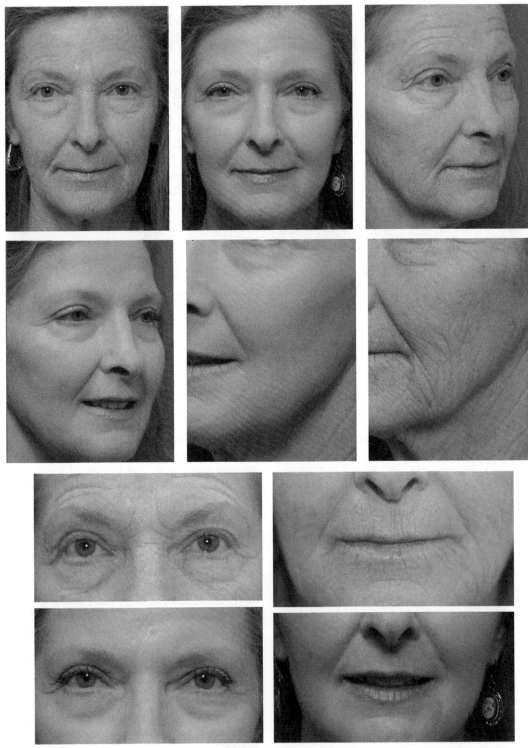

Fig. 23. Left, this 61 year old woman is a classic example of negative skin aging due to sun damage and long-term smoking; her structural changes are mild; therefore, a facelift would not be a first choice. She has prominent perioral and periorbital wrinkles, blotchy pigment throughout and thick, opaque skin. Right, the changes 6 months after peeling alone clearly show the power of this technique. The overall appearance is bright and healthy. She has a look of youth that was not present before. The wrinkles around the mouth and upper face have been nicely eradicated without depigmentation. Note the skin tightening, shrinking of upper lid skin, and shortening of upper lip. The improvement of skin quality of the mid-face is quite dramatic.

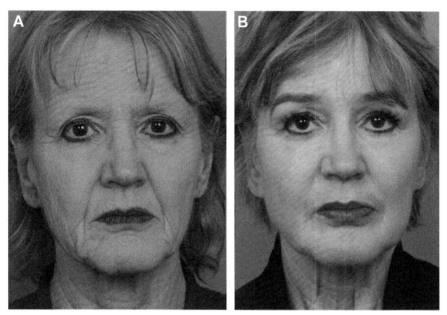

Fig. 24. (*A*) This 70 year old woman shows considerable facial wrinkling, but also generalized deflation which is a prominent feature of her appearance. (*B*) Results 14 months after lipofilling and croton oil peeling. This synergistic combination has the potential of providing a greater aesthetic impact than a facelift.

cause hypopigmentation. In general, this hypopigmentation is well worth it and does not have the artificial, porcelain look of the older peels. Careful assessment preoperatively is important because there are patients who have lighter upper lip skin naturally which may become more obvious once the solar damage is improved. Also, it is prudent to point out to the patient if there is hypopigmentation due to previous dermabrasion or carbon dioxide lasers treatment.

Sun exposure in the early recovery can result in hyperpigmentation, usually in dark skinned individuals. Strict sun avoidance in the first 2 weeks along with pretreatment to suppress melanocytes is important. After the first 2 weeks, most patients can tolerate a physical sun block resulting in considerably more freedom. Hyperpigmentation

can be treated with tretinoin and hydroquinone 4%, but it can look blotchy and linger for a few weeks.

A herpetic infection is a constant fear; therefore, all patients are treated prophylactically with valacyclovir 500 mg twice a day starting 3 days prior to the peel and continuing for 7 days after. If an outbreak is suspected, the dose of the antiviral is doubled and a topical antiviral such as penciclovir is used. This is carefully applied with a cotton-tipped applicator so as not to spread the infection.

As has been discussed, the potential of spreading genital herpes to the face can be very troubling. All patients must be considered potential carriers so they need to be warned to wash their hands before touching their face when allowed on day 8. To date, we have seen no

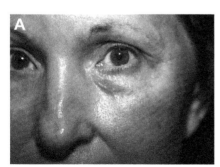
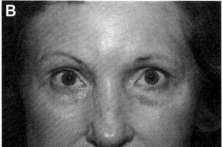

Fig. 25. (*A*) Early skin thickening or scar. (*B*) Result after one injection of intralesional 5-FU.

herpetic infection since switching to the bismuth paste and a no-touch technique.

Milia were common when occlusive ointments were used; they are much less frequent with the bismuth mask. Milia can be treated with tretinoin (after 6 weeks) or carefully excised with a fine needle.

Erythema lasting more than 12 weeks is possible, but it always subsides completely and has not required treatment as was sometimes needed with ablative CO_2 lasers. There has been a notable decrease in erythema since the use of taping and bismuth subgallate paste.

SUMMARY

The finding that croton oil is the critical peeling ingredient has been pivotal in the evolution of deep chemical peeling. By modulating the croton oil concentration, the process has been slowed, giving the surgeon control of the peel; by using appropriate application technique, the desired clinical result is possible without causing hypopigmentation. By lowering the croton oil concentration, now surgeons have a controllable option for effective skin resurfacing.

Peeling older patients with established wrinkles is an obvious indication for croton oil peels and peeling younger patients incrementally to keep up with aging is an interesting prospect that opens up these peels to a much wider audience. The prevention and potential treatment of non-melanoma skin cancer is an intriguing proposition that deserves more interest and research.

Although laser resurfacing, especially erbium, is a viable alternative, there are cellular differences. Laser resurfacing results in increased collagen but elastin is not elicited. The clinical observation is that erbium laser simply does not improve perioral lines and chin wrinkles like croton oil peels. Lased skin is thinner and there is a degradation of results after a few years. The surprising stability of results, if not permanence, is a hallmark of croton oil peels.

When discussing laser versus peels, the very high cost of lasers must be considered. With the insignificant cost of peels, it is my belief that lasers would have to be much better to justify recommending them. One of the main purposes of this article is to give readers practical guidance to try these peels before spending large sums on a laser.

REFERENCES

1. Hetter GP. An examination of the phenol-croton oil peel:part 1. Dissecting the formula. Plast Reconstr Surg 2000;105:227–39.
2. Bensimon RH. Croton oil peels. Aesthet Surg J 2008; 28:33–45.
3. Hetter GP. An examination of the phenol-croton oil peel: Part IV. Face peel results with different concentrations of phenol and croton oil. Plast Reconstr Surg 2000;105:1061–83.
4. Bensimon RH. Technical use of croton oil peels. In: Tonnard PL, Verpaele AM, Bensimon RH, editors. Centrofacial rejuvenation. New York: Thieme Publishers; 2018. p. 330.
5. Kaminaka C, Yamamoto Y, Yonei N, et al. Phenol peels as a novel therapeutic approach for actinic keratosis and bowen disease: prospective pilot trial with assessment of clinical histological and immunohistochemical correlations. J Am Acad Dermatol 2009;60:615–25.
6. Kaminaka C, Yamamoto Y, Furukawa F. Nevoid basal cell carcinoma syndrome successfully treated with trichloroacetic acid and phenol peeling. J Dermatol 2007;34:841–3.
7. Hantash BM, Stewart DB, Cooper ZA, et al. Facial resurfacing for non-melanoma skin cancer prophylaxis. Arch Dermatol 2006;142:976–82.

Radiofrequency Microneedling

Macrene Alexiades, MD, PhD[a,b,*]

KEYWORDS

- Radiofrequency • Microneedling • Laxity • Rhytids • Energy-based devices • Lasers • Cellulite

KEY POINTS

- Radiofrequency devices are energy-based tools applied as cutaneous treatment of the face and body.
- Microneedle electrode delivery of radiofrequency is an advance that has provided temperature and impedance measurements and improved targeting of dermal and subcutaneous tissues.
- Radiofrequency microneedling has improved treatment efficacy and expanded indications in skin rejuvenation, rhytids, laxity, acne scars and cellulite.

BACKGROUND

The application of energy-based devices such as radiofrequency (RF) for the treatment of skin laxity has advanced during the past 2 decades, most recently with the development of RF microneedling.[1–3] Skin laxity, described as sagging of the skin and attributed to loss in elastin, is one of the primary findings in skin aging (**Table 1**).[4,5] A survey by the American Society for Dermatologic Surgery revealed that.[6] Although the gold standard treatment of facial and neck laxity continues to be surgical rhytidectomy, demand is high for nonsurgical alternatives that avoid the risks of anesthesia, postsurgical morbidity, and the potential of an unnatural cosmetic outcome. Microneedle delivery of RF has resulted in clinically meaningful outcomes in cases of mild-to-moderate skin laxity and cellulite with the advantages of favorable recovery and side effect profile.

Clinical Presentation

Candidates for RF microneedling include patients presenting with mild-to-moderate skin laxity of the facial or neck skin or with cellulite or rhytids on the body. Skin sagging, crepiness, or loose skin to the face or neck are the clinical findings of *skin laxity* (see **Table 1**). Deepening facial creases, jowls, lines, or folding on face and/or body are findings most associated with *rhytids*. Linear indentations, dimples, and contour irregularity to the buttocks or thighs are the clinical criteria for *cellulite* (**Table 2**).[7]

Diagnosis and Grading

In rendering a diagnosis of rhytids, laxity, or skin aging of the face and neck, it is recommended to use a validated skin aging classification and document a baseline grade for each category (see **Table 1**).[1–5] The gradation of skin laxity findings on face include nasolabial folds, melolabial folds, jowels, submental and submandibular folds, and neck platysmal strands.[4,5] Loss of elasticity and recoil are clinical findings that may be independently tested using elastometry measurements.[2,3]

Body skin rhytids, laxity, and cellulite have been assessed by the presence or absence of surface irregularities including dimples and linear indentations.[7–9] Cellulite grading scales have been tested and used including the Alexiades Cellulite scale.[7–9]

Mechanism of Action

During the third decade of life, skin composition typically begins to deteriorate. Collagen and elastin synthesis decrease, whereas elastin fibers undergo degradation secondary to sun exposure.[10–14] The elasticity and resilience of the skin are attributed to the elastic fiber system, which

^a Yale University School of Medicine, New Haven, CT, USA; ^b Dermatology & Laser Surgery Center of New York, NY, USA
* Dermatology & Laser Surgery Center of New York, 955 Park Avenue, New York, NY 10028.
E-mail address: drmacrene@nyderm.org

Facial Plast Surg Clin N Am 31 (2023) 495–502
https://doi.org/10.1016/j.fsc.2023.06.010

Table 1
Alexiades skin aging scale

Grading Scale	Descriptive Parameter	Categories of Skin Aging and Photo Damage							Overall Score	Patient Satisfaction (Y/N)
		Rhytides	Laxity	Elastosis	Dyschromia	Erythema Telangiectasia	Keratoses	Texture		
0	None	None	None	None	None	None	None	None		
1	Mild	Wrinkles in motion, few, superficial	Localized to NL folds	Early, minimal yellow hue	Few (1–3) discrete small (<5 mm) lentigines	Pink E or few T, localized to single site	Few	Subtle irregularity		
1.5	Mild	Wrinkles in motion, multiple, superficial	Localized NL and early ML folds	Yellow hue of early, localized PO EB	Several (3–6), discrete small lentigines	Pink E or several T localized to 2 sites	Several	Mild irregularity in few areas		
2	Moderate	Wrinkles at rest, few, localized, superficial	Localized, NL/ML folds, early jowels, early submental/SM	Yellow hue, localized PO EB	Multiple (7–10), small lentigines	Red E or multiple T localized to 2 sites	Multiple small	Rough in few, localized sites		
2.5	Moderate	Wrinkles at rest, multiple, localized, superficial	Localized, prominent NL/ML folds, jowels and SM	Yellow hue, PO and malar EB	Multiple, small and few large lentigines	Red E or multiple T, localized to 3 sites	Multiple large	Rough in several localized areas		
3	Advanced	Wrinkles at rest, multiple, PO and forehead, PO and perioral sites, superficial	Prominent NL/ML folds, jowels and SM, early neck strands	Yellow hue, EB involving PO, malar, and other sites	Many (10–20) small and large lentigines	Violaceous E or many T, multiple sites	Many	Rough in multiple, localized sites		

3.5	Advanced	Wrinkles at rest, multiple, generalized, superficial; few, deep	Deep NL/ML folds, prominent jowels and SM, prominent neck strands	Deep yellow hue, extensive EB with little uninvolved skin	Numerous (>20) or multiple large with little uninvolved skin	Violaceous E, numerous T, little uninvolved skin	Little uninvolved skin	Mostly rough, little uninvolved skin
4	Severe	Wrinkles throughout, numerous, extensively distributed, deep	Marked NL/ML folds, jowels and SM, neck redundancy and strands	Deep yellow hue EB throughout, comedones	Numerous, extensive, no uninvolved skin	Deep, violaceous E, numerous T throughout	No uninvolved skin	Rough throughout

Abbreviations: E, erythema; EB, elastotic beads; ML, melolabial; NL, nasolabial; PO, periorbital; SM, submandibular; T, telangiectasia.

Republished with permission from Alexiades-Armenakas M. A quantitative and comprehensive grading scale for rhytides, laxity, and photoaging. J Drugs Dermatol. 2006 Sep;5(8):808-9. PMID: 16989197; Alexiades-Armenakas M. Rhytides, laxity, and photoaging treated with a combination of radiofrequency, diode laser, and pulsed light and assessed with a comprehensive grading scale. J Drugs Dermatol. 2006 Sep;5(8):731-8. PMID: 16989187.

confers the deformability and passive recoil of tissue.[12] In contrast, collagen fibers provide tensile strength. Finally, hyaluronic acid, a humectant, provides turgor and skin moisture. Genetic alterations in elastic fibers are associated with sagging skin and loss of recoil, elasticity, and resilience[10–14] (see **Table 2**).

The mechanism of action of RF in skin rejuvenation has been investigated by the author and others during the past 2 decades. RF, composed of 3 kHz to 24 GHz frequencies, and delivered as an oscillating electrical current, induces collisions and rotations of charged and polar atoms and molecules in tissue.[1,15] Heat is generated from the resistance of tissue components to the movement of charged and polar molecules within the oscillating RF field. This resistance, termed impedance, generates heat relative to the amount of current and time, converting electrical current to thermal energy.[1,15]

RF skin heating at a specified target temperature range defined by the author results in partial denaturation of collagen and dermal structures resulting in histologic dermal remodeling and correlating with clinical rhytid and laxity reduction.[1–5,15] RF delivery results in increased collagen, elastin and hyaluronic acid, which correlates clinically with improvements in the smoothness and elastic properties of the skin.[1–5,15] The author discovered that the cohort treated with target temperatures of greater than 70°C, which results in complete collagen denaturation, correlated with less clinical improvement as compared with the cohort treated with intradermal temperatures of 62°C to 67°C, which results in partially denatured collagen and correlated with superior clinical outcomes.[3,15] The author has published her theory postulating that heat-induced partially denatured collagens reveal RGD or arginylglycylaspartic acid; the important cell adhesion motif signals a cascade of neocollagenesis and neoelastinogenesis.[3,15] This dermal remodeling process continues up to 12 months following treatment correlating with progressive clinical improvement correlating clinically with clinical rhytid and laxity reduction.[1–5,15]

Radiofrequency Subtypes

RF devices may be classified as skin surface applied (noninvasive) and needle or probe-delivered (minimally invasive) the latter being the subject of this article.[1] RF microneedling may be classified according to electrode configuration: monopolar RF uses a single electrode and a grounding pad and bipolar uses opposing electrode pairs in the handpiece tip wherein the current traverses the skin via a closed circuit. Although the penetration depth of skin surface-applied RF is approximately one-half the distance between the electrodes, microneedle RF delivery bypasses this barrier to deliver energy directly into the dermis and subcutis. The breakthrough of the first RF microneedling device (Profound, Candela, Wayland, MA) included thermistors in the microneedle tips permitting real-time feedback of impedance and temperature.[2]

The penetration depth depends on needle quality, mechanics of deployment, bevel edge, skin hydration and other factors, electrode configuration, and anatomic location. Once RF is deployed within the tissue, structures with higher conductivity and impedance generate more heat: fat, bone, and dry skin have low conductivities such that current flows around rather than through these structures; hydrated skin possesses high electrical conductivity via the effects of water dipole moment, thus

---

Table 2
Alexiades cellulite scale

Grade	Contour	Dimple Density	Dimple Distribution	Dimple Depth	Diameter % Change
0	Smooth	0	0	0	$100 \times \{[\text{pre-post}]/\text{pre}\}$
1	1 indents	1–2/site	1 site	Shallow (1–2 mm)	
2	2 indents	3–5/site	2 sites	Moderate (3–4 mm)	
3	3 indents	6–8/site	3 sites	Advanced (5–6 mm)	
4	>3 indents	>9/site	4 or more sites	Deep (>7 mm)	

Contour. 0 = smooth; 1 = one indentation; 2 = 2 indentations; 3 = 3 indentations; and 4 = 4 or more indentations; indent = overall indentation of contour to thigh. *Density*: 0 = none; 1 = 1–2 per site; 2 = 3–5 per site; 3 = 6–8 peer site; and 4 = 9–10 or more per site. Sites (graded individually): buttock, anterior thigh upper, anterior thigh lower, posterior thigh upper, posterior thigh lower; upper refers to upper half and lower refers to lower half of thigh length. *Distribution:* 0 = none, 1 = 1site; 2 = 2 sites; 3 = 3 sites; and 4 = 4 or more sites. *Depth:* 0 = n/a; 1 = shallow (1–2 mm); 2 = moderate (3–4 mm); 3 = advanced (5–6 mm); and 4 = deep (≥7 mm in depth). Dimple depth was estimated in the blinded evaluations of photographs. *Diameter:* mean difference in diameter (mm) on photographic superimposition.

Adapted from Alexiades-Armenakas, Macrene, Dover, Jeffrey S. and Arndt, Kenneth A.(2008) Unipolar radiofrequency treatment to improve the appearance of cellulite',Journal of Cosmetic and Laser Therapy,10:3,148 — 153 To link to this Article: https://doi.org/10.1080/14764170802279651 URL: https://doi.org/10.1080/14764170802279651.

allowing greater penetration of current (Alexiades, 2023, unpublished data).

Monopolar Radiofrequency Microneedling

Voluderm, Lumenis, Israel

An RF microneedling device delivers uninsulated microneedle electrodes that are grounded to the pad in the handpiece tip to create a closed loop (Voluderm, Lumenis, Israel). The RF current is delivered via a tip composed of an array of 36 microneedles that penetrate the treated area as the needle temperature increases, resulting in a treatment that does not require topical or local anesthesia. The full-length heating of the needles, which come in 0.6 and 1 mm length, results in heating of both dermal and epidermal layers but superficially penetrating into dermis, resulting in textural improvements[16] (Alexiades, article in preparation).

Intracel, Jeisys, Korea

Another variation is the Intracel (Jeisys Medical, Korea) device where the grounding pad is applied to the patient's lumbar region. Here, it is postulated that conductive heating extends the zone of treatment distal to the microneedle tips that penetrate at increments up to 2.0 mm in depth. Efficacy in the treatment of acne scars has been reported.[17]

Bipolar Radiofrequency Microneedling

Profound, Candela, Wayland, MA

In 2010, the author and others attained Federal Drug Administration (FDA) clearance for the first needle-delivered bipolar RF (Profound, Candela, Wayland, MA).[2,3] The first device to deliver RF via a microneedle electrode array directly into the reticular dermis, the Profound bypassed the epidermis and papillary dermis, measuring for

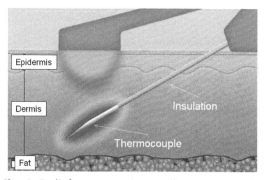

Fig. 1. Radiofrequency microneedle prototype. The first device delivered microneedle electrodes into the dermis with thermistors at the needle tips and contact cooling at the surface. In most models, the distal microneedle is exposed and proximal portion insulated to protect the epidermis.

the first time in situ real-time impedance and temperature using thermistors in the electrode tips (**Fig. 1**). This device has been updated and advanced in needle configuration, gauge, manufacturing, and protocol refinements. Single-use treatment cartridges deliver 5 pairs of independently controlled, 32-gauge, bipolar 250 μm microneedles spaced 1.25 mm apart; each needle pair is independently sensed and powered by the RF generator. The proximal 3 mm of the 6 mm needle is insulated to protect the superficial portion of the skin during treatment, whereas the distal 3 mm length is exposed to allow electrical current flow between needle pairs to generate 3-dimensional zones of thermal effects in the target. The dermal handpiece is at a 25° angle so that the tips of the needles are at a 2 mm depth from the epidermis. Current flows between each needle pair resulting in fractionated zones (one between each pair) of thermal injury situated in the dermis 2 mm from the surface of the skin. Epidermal cooling is achieved via an integrated thermokinetic cooling bar on the applicator. Intradermal targeting is ensured by impedance measurements in the needle tips and software ensuring firing within a specified impedance range. A target temperature is selected by the user and energy is delivered until the target temperature is attained and energy titrated to maintain precise target temperature for a selected pulse duration.[2,3] The subcutaneous handpiece delivers bipolar RF pulses using 5 pairs of microneedle electrodes deployed into the dermis at an angle of 75° with the exposed portion extending from 3.9 to 5.8 mm beneath the skin surface (Profound Sub-Q, Candela, Wayland, MA).[8,9] Zones of thermal injury with real-time temperature monitoring using temperature sensors in each electrode tip maintain a preselected target temperature regardless of varying skin conditions and improving consistency between patients.

The author and colleagues compared baseline and 3 to 6-month follow-up photographs of 15 patients who underwent skin tightening using a microneedle RF device with those of 6 patients who had undergone rhytidectomy.[2] The RF device patients were judged to have a 16% improvement from baseline and the surgical patients were judged to have a 49% improvement from baseline laxity grades, or a 0.46 versus 1.20 laxity grade reduction, respectively. The laxity grade reduction resulting from a single microneedle RF treatment was 37% that of a surgical facelift.[2] In the subsequent multicenter clinical trial and multiarm studies of target dermal temperatures ranging from 52°C to 78°C, the current author and colleagues discovered that temperatures 67°C cohort resulted in maximal neocollagenesis, neoelastogenesis and hyaluronic acid production and correlated clinically with maximal rhytid and laxity reduction and a 100% response rate.[3] Higher and lower target temperatures demonstrated less efficacy. The findings using needle-delivered RF support the theory that partially denatured collagen is more effective at triggering a strong wound healing response.[15] **Fig. 2** shows 2 sets of before and after photographs following a single microneedle RF treatment (Profound, Candela, Wayland, MA). Arrows indicate findings of laxity at baseline including jowels and submental laxity at baseline and the significant reduction of jowels and submental laxity with the restoration of mandibular definition on follow-up after a single treatment. Similar skin tightening effects were observed on body skin laxity when the subcutaneous handpiece was used to treat cellulite.[8,9] When treating with microneedle RF on the body skin, a reduction in linear undulations and textural irregularities were observed.[8,9]

A recent variation to the system called the Profound Matrix involves vertical insertion of microneedle RF electrodes to up to 3 insertion depths. An array of 49 (7 × 7) ultra-thin semiinsulated microelectrode chamfered needles, with a diameter of 0.16 mm (34 gauge) may be inserted up to 7 mm deep with intervals of 0.8 mm at up to 3 insertion depths. This multidepth insertion and treatment allows for a greater zone of coagulation and may improve outcomes for pathologies requiring larger zones of dermal treatment (Alexiades, article in preparation).

Morpheus, InMode, Israel

Adjustable-depth and multidepth targeting are 2 key technological advancements in RF microneedling that enable delivering energy to different depths depending on condition and anatomic site, and multiple depths on a single insertion,

respectively. The first system to pioneer both features (Morpheus8, InMode, Israel) enables the user to program and target up to 7 mm deep at 1 mm increments and up to 3 different depths per insertion.[16,18] Earlier versions of this device (Fractora, Invasix, Israel) administered 1 MHz to RF-conducting needles, alternating current with 2 long side electrodes. The handpiece cartridges come as 600 or 3000 μm long needles, which are 200 × 300 μm wide at the base, for middermal and deep dermal or subdermal delivery, respectively. The middermal delivers 60 microneedles while the full dermal or deep dermal/subdermal handpiece contains 24 uncoated or coated needles, respectively. The handpiece is loaded to the FractoraTM platform (also applicable to InModeTM or BodyTiteTM platforms, Invasix Ltd./ InMode MD Ltd., Israel). The device has been reported to result in significant improvement in acne and acne scars.[16]

Infini/Genius, Lutronic, Billerica, MA

A device that allows for adjustable needle depths to 0.5, 1.0, 1.5, 2.0, and 3.5 mm (Infini, Lutronic offers a 49-needle tip [10 mm × 10 mm, 7 × 7 needles] and a 16-needle tip [5 mm × 5 mm, 4 × 4 needles]).[17] The microneedles are surgical stainless steel gold-coated for conductivity and then double coated with an insulating silicon compound, except for the distal 300-μm tip. The needles have a diameter of 200 μm and point diameter of 20 μm. Insulation of the proximal portions of the needles restrict the treatment zone to the distal tip, and protects the epidermis from electrothermal injury. Clinical trials have demonstrated wrinkle reduction following treatment with this device, with clinician-assessed overall efficacy and patient satisfaction index are similar at from 80.7% to 88.9% and 81.3% to 85.9%, respectively.[17] Although the system lacks real-

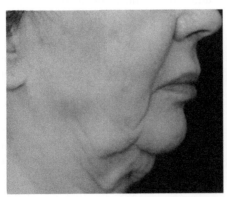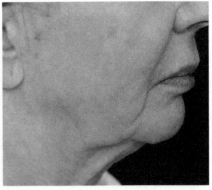

Fig. 2. Before and after images of radiofrequency microneedling using the Profound system. Following a single treatment, clinically significant improvement in skin laxity is observed during a 6-month follow-up interval.

time temperature feedback, it has incorporated impedance measurements.

Intensif, EndyMed, Israel

Another bipolar microneedle RF device (Intensif, EndyMed Medical, Caesarea, Israel) includes 25 noninsulated gold-plated microneedle electrodes 300 μm in diameter at the base gradually tapering to a sharp edge. Penetration depth of up to 3.5 mm may be administered at 0.1 mm digitally controlled increments.[19] Maximal power is 25 W with a maximal pulse duration is 200 milliseconds. The electrical impedance difference between the epidermis (high) and the dermis (low) ensures RF flow through the dermis. The RF emission delivered throughout the length of the needle results in effective coagulation with minimal or no bleeding, and dermal heating.[19]

SUMMARY

RF microneedling is a significant technological advance that has demonstrated clinical improvements in rhytids, laxity, skin texture, and cellulite. Direct in situ delivery, impedance measurements, temperature measurements, energy delivery controls, and targeting of various skin depths have improved tissue targeting have correlated with improved outcomes. RF delivery through microneedle insertion allows for relatively precise penetration depths, real-time temperature, and impedance measurements and multidepth targeting.

CLINICS CARE POINTS

- When treating with RF microneedling, it is critical to ensure complete needle penetration and insertion into the skin.
- Incomplete needle insertion may result in epidermal injury and reduces treatment depth.
- For most RF microneedling devices, adequate topical and/or local anaesthesia is advised to improve treatment comfort for the patient.
- In the case of devices which lack real-time feedback of tissue temperature or impedance, ensure the needle depth and energy delivered is correct for the treatment area and indication.

REFERENCES

1. Alexiades M. Microneedle radiofrequency. Facial Plast Surg Clin North Am 2020;28(1):9–15.

2. Alexiades-Armenakas M, Rosenberg D, Renton B, et al. Blinded, randomized, quantitative grading comparison of minimally invasive, fractional RF and surgical face-lift to treat skin laxity. Arch Dermatol 2010;146:396–405.

3. Alexiades-Armenakas M, Newman J, Willey A, et al. Prospective multicenter clinical trial of a minimally-invasive temperature-controlled bipolar fractional RF system for rhytid and laxity treatment. Dermatol Surg 2013;39(2):263–73.

4. Alexiades-Armenakas M. A quantitative and comprehensive grading scale for rhytides, laxity, and photoaging. J Drugs Dermatol 2006;5(8):808–9. PMID: 16989197.

5. Alexiades-Armenakas M. Rhytides, laxity, and photoaging treated with a combination of radiofrequency, diode laser, and pulsed light and assessed with a comprehensive grading scale. J Drugs Dermatol 2006;5(8):731–8. PMID: 16989187.

6. American Society for Dermatologic Surgery (ASDS) 2021 Consumer Survey on Cosmetic Dermatologic Procedures. Available at: https://www.asds.net/portals/0/PDF/consumer-survey-2021-infographic.pdf.

7. Alexiades-Armenakas M, Dover J, Arndt K. Unipolar radiofrequency treatment to improve the appearance of cellulite'. J Cosmet Laser Ther 2008;10(3):148–53.

8. Alexiades M, Munavalli G, Goldberg D, et al. Prospective multicenter clinical trial of a temperature-controlled subcutaneous microneedle fractional bipolar RF system for the treatment of cellulite. Dermatol Surg 2018;44(10):1262–71.

9. Alexiades M, Munavalli GS. Single treatment protocol with microneedle fractional radiofrequency for treatment of body skin laxity and fat deposits. Lasers Surg Med 2021;53(8):1026–31.

10. El-Domyati M, Attia S, Saleh F, et al. Intrinsic aging vs. photoaging: a comparative histopathological, immunohistochemical, and ultrastructural study of skin. Exp Dermatol 2002;11:398–405.

11. Heinz A. Elastic fibers during aging and disease. Ageing Res Rev 2021;66:101255.

12. Kielty CM, Sherratt MJ, Shuttleworth CA. Elastic fibres. J Cell Sci 2002;115:2817–28.

13. Lewis KG, Bercovitch L, Dill SW, et al. Acquired disorders of elastic tissue: part I. Increased elastic tissue and solar elastotic syndromes. J Am Acad Dermatol 2004;51:1–21.

14. Lewis KG, Bercovitch L, Dill SW, et al. Acquired disorders of elastic tissue: Part II. decreased elastic tissue. J Am Acad Dermatol 2004;51:165–85.

15. Alexiades M, Berube D. Randomized, blinded, 3-arm clinical trial assessing optimal temperature and duration for treatment with minimally invasive fractional RF. Dermatol Surg 2015;41(5):623–32.

16. Kauvar ANB, Gershonowitz A. Clinical and histologic evaluation of a fractional radiofrequency treatment of wrinkles and skin texture with novel 1-mm long ultra-thin electrode pins. Lasers Surg Med 2022; 54(1):54–61.

17. Calderhead RG, Goo BL, Lauro F, et al. The Clinical Efficacy And Safety Of Microneedling Fractional RF In The Treatment Of Facial Wrinkles: A Multicenter Study With The Infini System In 499 Patients. 2013 White paper, us.aesthetic.lutronic.com.

18. Dayan E, Chia C, Burns AJ, et al. Adjustable depth fractional radiofrequency combined with bipolar radiofrequency: a minimally invasive combination treatment for skin laxity. Aesthet Surg J 2019; 39(Suppl_3):S112–9.

19. Kaplan H, Kaplan L. Combination of microneedle radiofrequency, fractional radiofrequency skin resurfacing and multi-source non-ablative skin tightening for minimal-downtime, full-face skin rejuvenation. J Cosmet Laser Ther 2016;18(8):438–41.

Ultrasound Therapy for the Skin

Anni Wong, MD[a], Anne S. Lowery, MD[b], Jason D. Bloom, MD[b,c,*]

KEYWORDS

- Ultrasound • Thermal injury zones • Facial rejuvenation • Noninvasive facial rejuvenation
- Skin laxity • Skin tightening • Skin lifting • Ulthera

KEY POINTS

- Ultrasound therapy is a nonsurgical skin rejuvenation procedure, which induces controlled thermal injury in the tissue, stimulating the wound-healing cascade and neocollagenesis.
- Ultrasound energy can be focused to reach deeper tissues, including the superficial muscle aponeurotic system while sparing the epidermis, allowing for tissue tightening in a plane deeper than other skin resurfacing modalities and avoiding adverse effects of epidermal disrupting techniques.
- The ideal patient has mild to moderate laxity of the skin, desire a "lifting" effect of the eyebrow, sub-mentum, and/or neck, and can be any Fitzpatrick skin type.
- Studies have demonstrated clinically significant improvement in brow lift and in skin laxity of the lower face and neck, with high patient-reported satisfaction.
- Treatments are well tolerated and adverse effects such as edema, erythema, ecchymosis, and post-inflammatory pigmentation are mild, short-lived, and self-limiting in nature.

INTRODUCTION

Various changes occur to the aging face, from textural and pigmentary changes to the development of wrinkles and loss of volume and skin elasticity. As patients search for facial rejuvenation options, there is an increasing demand for less invasive and effective modalities with decreased recovery time. As such, the use of injectables and energy-based devices has become ever more popular. Although injectable neurotoxins and dermal fillers are most frequently used and help address dynamic rhytids and volume losses of aging, these options have little effect on skin laxity or rejuvenation.[1] In an attempt to close this gap, there has been an influx of minimally invasive skin rejuvenation treatments, broadly categorized as ablative skin resurfacing (ASR) or non-ablative skin rejuvenation (NSR).[2] In general, rejuvenation by these modalities works by inducing thermal injury to the tissue to stimulate a wound healing response and subsequent collagen remodeling and contraction.

ASR modalities such as carbon dioxide (CO_2) and erbium-doped yttrium aluminum garnet (YAG) lasers and treatments such as deep chemical peel and dermabrasion have been time-tested to provide significant results in treating superficial rhytides of the aging face. ASR options also target and ablate the epidermis, allowing for reepithelization and neocollagenesis. Subsequently, its use can be associated with prolonged and uncomfortable postoperative recovery as well as risk of scarring, infection, and pigment changes.[3] In addition, it is not for all skin types.

NSR alternatives work by selectively inducing controlled thermal injury within the dermis, but spare the overlying epidermis thus avoiding the

[a] Department of Otorhinolaryngology-Head and Neck Surgery, University of Pennsylvania, 3737 Market Street, Suite 302, Philadelphia, PA 19104, USA; [b] Department of Otorhinolaryngology-Head and Neck Surgery, University of Pennsylvania, 3400 Spruce Street, Philadelphia, PA 19104, USA; [c] Bloom Facial Plastic Surgery, Two Town Place, Suite 110, Bryn Mawr, PA 19010, USA
* Corresponding author.
E-mail address: DrJBloom@bloomfps.com

Facial Plast Surg Clin N Am 31 (2023) 503–510
https://doi.org/10.1016/j.fsc.2023.05.008

undesirable post-procedural effects seen with epidermal disrupting techniques.[2] NSR modalities include options such as intense pulsed light, pulse dye laser, neodymium:YAG, radiofrequency (RF) heating. Although the rate of adverse effects is lowest with non-ablative options, improvements are often modest, inconsistent, and often require serial treatments over a 6 to 12 month period.[4]

To continue to meet the demand for a minimally invasive skin rejuvenation that also offers effective and consistent results, ultrasound as an energy modality for esthetic application soon entered the playing field as an NSR alterative. Similar to other NSR energy-based devices, therapeutic ultrasound also works on the premise of creating thermal injury to stimulate new collagen formation, leading to tightening and lifting of the skin. However, ultrasound energy can be tightly focused and offers deeper penetration in the tissue which allows higher temperatures to be reached, without injury to the more superficial tissues. Because of this, it has been found to be superior to other skin tightening technologies.[5]

ULTRASOUND AS THERAPEUTIC MODALITY AND MECHANISM OF ACTION

Ultrasound energy is focused to a point in the tissue, generating molecular vibration leading to heat formation, up to 60°C to 65°C. At this temperature, collagen denatures followed by neocollagenesis.[6] Coagulative changes to the tissue occur within the focal region of the beam creating a well-defined thermal injury zone (TIZ) or thermal coagulation point (TCP).[7] The focal injured tissue undergoes the wound healing cascade with tissue contracture and collagen remodeling, leading to tightening and lifting of the skin. Suh and colleagues observed that dermal collagen and elastic fibers were regenerated in increased numbers and rearranged resulting in thickening of the reticular dermis and uninterrupted epidermis.[4] Clinical effect of the tissue remodeling may be seen by 3 months and results can last for about 1 year.[7,8]

High-intensity focused ultrasound (HIFU) has been used for the treatment of benign prostate hypertrophy and tumors of the liver, prostate, uterus, breast, and kidney. Its mechanism is through inducing tissue damage both by thermal injury and the cavitation process. In the esthetic arena, HIFU has been used for lipolysis, using both thermal action to cause adipocyte apoptosis and ultrasonic mechanical fat destruction through cavitation.[9] For facial esthetic use such as skin tightening and lifting, microfocused ultrasound (MFUS) is applied. Unlike HIFU, MFUS only uses the thermal effect due to lower levels of focused

ultrasound energy per unit area (0.4–1.2 J/mm²), higher frequencies (from 4 to 19 MHz), shorter pulse durations (50–200 ms), and focal depths of 1.5 to 4.5 mm.[4,9,10]

With these parameters of MFUS, energy can be precisely focused so a microscopically small volume of tissue (<1 mm³) can be thermally ablated, leaving surrounding tissue uninjured. This is in contrast to other thermal ablation techniques such as RF, where there is a volumetric heating effect with diffuse energy delivered to the dermis, but can also travel along connective tissue into the subdermis.[4,11] Rather than creating a macroscopic region of ablation, MFUS creates an array of focal damage with a segment of untreated tissue between two TCPs. Analogous to the concept of fractional ablative laser, the bridging undamaged tissue allows for a rapid healing response to the adjacent thermally injured areas.[4,12]

There are several other advantages of MFUS as an NSR alternative. Because MFUS uses a sharp focus of ultrasound beam into the tissue, the power density of the converging beams is much lower as it passes through the epidermis than its focal point. Consequently, there are minimal energy absorption and tissue heating at the epidermal level. This not only leaves the epidermis undamaged but also avoids the need for any skin cooling for epidermal protection that is often required for other energy-based devices that cause unexpected thermal changes within the skin.[12] Its tight focus of energy is also able to reach subdermal tissue of greater depths, such as the superficial muscle aponeurotic system (SMAS), allowing for tissue tightening in a plane deeper than other types of devices.[13] Last, the absorption of ultrasound energy is independent of chromophores or melanin content of the skin. Its absorption is instead determined by the microscopic and bulk mechanical properties of tissue.[12] Because ultrasound therapy does not target melanin or chromophores, it carries a lower risk of pigmentary changes in dark skin types compared with photo-based energy sources[9] and is safe for all skin types.[4,9,11] In a study of 49 Asian patients with Fitzpatrick skin types III and IV by Chan and colleagues, two patients experienced post-inflammatory hyperpigmentation, which fully resolved within 9 months of treatment.[14]

Intense ultrasound beam (IUB) is another ultrasound technology that has recently come into the esthetics market. Unlike MFUS which creates an elongated pinpoint TIZ perpendicular to the skin surface, IUB creates an elongated 3-dimensional (3D) cylindrically shaped TIZ parallel to the skin surface. The TIZ lies parallel to the direction of the collagen fibers, and therefore, the ensuing collagen contraction creates vector lines of tightening along the direction of facial lines and wrinkles. Because of the geometric, volumetric cylinder shape of the beam, it generates fractional volumetric and directional thermal coagulation of the tissue.[15,16]

DEVICE TECHNOLOGY

The Ulthera system (Ulthera, Inc, Mesa, AZ) is MFUS technology that received Food and Drug Administration (FDA) approval for noninvasive eyebrow lift in 2009, submental and neck lift in 2012, and the improvement of lines and wrinkles of the décolleté in 2014.

The Ulthera system consists of a control unit, a central processer with monitor, and a handpiece with four interchangeable transducers. The handpiece is dual functioning with a transducer capable of high-resolution ultrasonography imaging, using lower energy ultrasound, to provide visualization of the targeted tissue up to a depth of 8 mm (**Fig. 1**). This allows for visualization of dermal and subcutaneous structures before initiation of energy delivery for enhanced safety.

The control unit allows for adjustment of power output, exposure time, length of exposure line, distance between exposure zones, and time delay after each exposure. The interchangeable transducers come with varying focal depths and frequencies.

- A 1.5-mm focus depth, 10 MHz (source energy 0.25 J), newest available transducer, which targets more superficial dermis
- A 3.0-mm focus depth, 7.5 MHz (source energy 0.4–0.63 J): targets dermis
- A 4.5-mm focus depth, 7.5 MHz (source energy 0.75–1.05 J): targets subdermal tissues, including SMAS
- A 4.5-mm focus depth, 4.4 MHz (source energy 0.75–1.2 J): targets subdermal tissues, including SMAS

Tissue penetrance and frequency are indirectly related. Therefore, the lower frequency of the 4 MHz transducer can provide a more robust and deeper treatment depth compared with the 7 MHz transducer at a 4.5 mm focus.[1] The 4 MHz transducer can be used for treatment of the deeper fibromuscular layer of the cheek and jawline. The 3.0 and 1.5 mm transducers deliver less energy and target the reticular dermis, allowing for more superficial treatments that can be used on more sensitive locations with thinner skin such as the forehead and temples.[1,6] Each firing of the device delivers energy in a 25 mm line, creating 17 to 22 TCPs, spaced 1.1 to 1.5 mm apart.[1] Multiple exposure lines are placed 2 to 4 mm apart.

The Sofwave system (Sofwave Medical, Inc, Tustin, CA) is another ultrasound device that has received FDA clearance for improvement of facial fine lines and wrinkles in 2019 and lifting of the eyebrow, submentum, and neck in 2021. It additionally has a new clearance for the treatment of cellulite in the lower body. The Sofwave device uses IUB or synchronous ultrasound parallel beam technology. The device handpiece consists of seven transducers, each 4.5 mm × 1 mm, delivering high-intensity, high-frequency ultrasound energy as seven parallel beams, creating an array of 3D cylindrically shaped TIZ in the mid-dermis (**Fig. 2**). These coagulated columns of tissue lie parallel to the skin surface along the long axis of the transducers and parallel to the direction of

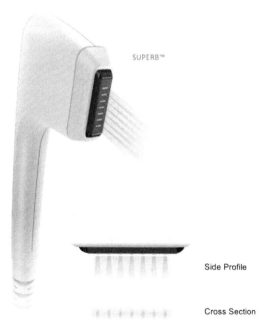

SUPERB™

Side Profile

Cross Section

Fig. 2. Sofwave handpiece with parallel beam technology. (Photo courtesy of Sofwave™.)

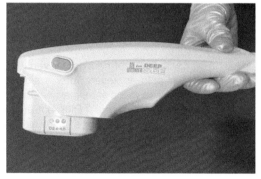

Fig. 1. Ulthera handpiece with interchangeable transducer (4 MHz, 4.5 mm treatment depth transducer shown). (Photo courtesy of Merz Aesthetics/Ulthera.)

the collagen fibers.[15] Most of the thermal effect is localized between 0.5 and 2 mm of the dermis, with treatment centered at a depth of 1.5 mm, thereby treating only the mid-dermal layer. Each pulse of Sofwave is equivalent to about 7 to 8 lines of Ulthera. Because of the volumetric effect of the beams, 28% of the mid-dermal tissue is covered in a single-treatment, two-pass procedure.

The handpiece also contains an integrated active cooling mechanism that continuously measures the skin temperature in real time to provide feedback-controlled skin cooling to protect the epidermal layer.[15,16]

Comparing Ulthera Versus Sofwave

The Ulthera system consists of multiple interchangeable hand pieces to target different tissue layers, whereas the Sofwave system consists of a single-hand piece to target a single-tissue layer, the mid-dermis. As such, the Ulthera device has ultrasound imaging to visualize and verify the appropriate targeted tissue layer and underlying deep structures as a safety measure to avoid injury to critical structures. In contrast, the Sofwave device does not have or require ultrasound imaging as its treatment is limited to a depth of 2 mm and therefore pose no risk of injury to underlying bone, fat, or nerves. Although both technologies boast minimal patient discomfort, Sofwave is less painful compared with Ulthera due to Sofwave's more superficial treatment depth. The ability to target the collagen-rich mid-dermal layer was not feasible with Ulthera until their release of the 1.5 mm transducer. With Ulthera, it should be noted that technique becomes more of a critical component when dealing with shallower tissue planes to prevent possible adverse effects.[17] Because of its synchronous beam technology and larger contact surface area of the probe, treatment times with Sofwave are shorter, approximately 30 to 45 minutes for the full face and neck.[15] Depending on the provider experience, patient tolerance, and treatment surface area, treatment times for full face and neck with Ulthera are generally less than 90 minutes (30–60 minutes for the face and 30–45 minutes for the neck).[8] In regard to pricing for the practice, Sofwave has pulse consumables, as price per pulse. Ulthera has a consumable fee for each transducer probe, where each probe has a useable lifespan of about 2100 lines and would require replacement after.

TECHNIQUE

Before treatment, the skin is cleaned, medicated with topical anesthetic, and the treatment areas defined and marked with a planning card. Treatment areas can include the cheek, periorbital areas (outside the orbital rim), brow, and neck. The depth of treatment and therefore selection of transducer to use for a specific area is determined by the skin thickness of the treatment site. Next, ultrasound gel is applied to the target site and the selected transducer is placed perpendicular and firmly to the skin. With the Ulthera device, the correct placement of the ultrasound probe is verified through ultrasound images on the monitor. The treatment is typically completed at two depths, with one pass of the 4.5 mm transducer for deeper penetration, followed by the 3 or 1.5 mm transducer for more superficial penetration.[18] With the exception of the infraorbital region, where the tissue is thin, treatment is completed only at the superficial focal depth.[1] The thyroid and the orbital area should be avoided.[6] A full-face treatment consists of 600 to 800 lines for best results.[7,8] With the Sofwave device, there is no verification with ultrasound imaging. Treatment similarly consists of two passes.

PATIENT SELECTION

As with any procedure, patient selection and establishing realistic expectations are important components of the treatment process. The ideal patient for noninvasive tissue tightening has mild to moderate laxity of the skin on the face and desire a "lifting" effect of the eyebrow, submentum, and/or neck. Patients who are concerned about risk and recovery and are willing to accept moderate efficacy in exchange for minimal risk are ideal candidates for non-ablative modalities. Factors such as the patient's age, extent of photodamage, and smoking may adversely affect collagen remodeling.[6] Younger patients tend to have greater results as they typically have a more robust healing response and better inherent skin elasticity.[1] Improved treatment outcomes have been shown to correlate with patient age, body mass index (BMI), skin type, and immune response.[9]

PRETREATMENT AND POSTTREATMENT

Pain associated with the treatment can be variable. Patient rated their pain as severe after a single-pass treatment in the absence of topical anesthetic in 54.4% of treatment sessions.[14] Different areas of the face have differing levels of sensitivity: the eyebrow and periorbital area were associated with greater pain (5.7 of 10) than that of the face (3.7 of 10) and neck (3.6 of 10).[19] In addition, the submental and submandibular areas are more sensitive than cheeks, possibly due to thinner tissue and proximity to bony prominences.[11]

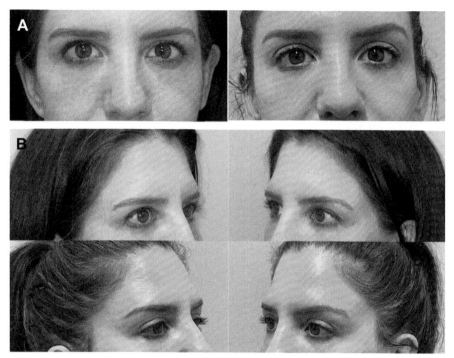

Fig. 3. A 45-year-old woman with eyebrow lift results from a single treatment of Sofwave at 6 weeks follow-up. (*A*) Before/after frontal images. (*B*) Before/after lateral images.

To enhance patient comfort, many methods have been attempted to mitigate pain, including oral nonsteroidal anti-inflammatory drugs (NSAIDs), acetaminophen, oral narcotics, oral anxiolytics, topical anesthetics, inhaled nitrous oxide and oxygen systems, anesthetic nerve blocks, and distraction techniques. In addition to oral NSAIDs or acetaminophen before treatment sessions, the lowest feasible energy setting should be used based on patient tolerance.[3] Topical lidocaine and narcotic analgesia were found to be superior to NSAIDs when user deeper transducers, but had no improvement in pain when using the 1.5 mm transducer.[20] One group shared that they have garnered positive patient experience with a combination of 30% topical lidocaine and oral ibuprofen or intramuscular ketorolac.[6]

After completion of the treatment, the ultrasound gel is cleaned and an emollient cream is applied.[6] Patients are typically educated on the expected posttreatment effects of mild erythema and edema and are discouraged from vigorous exercise for 3 to 5 days.[21] Any evidence of edema from the treatment typically subsided within 7 to 10 days.[11] Patients may resume their normal skincare regimens, and no specific aftercare is needed.

COMPLICATIONS

Pain associated with treatments is the most commonly reported adverse effect associated

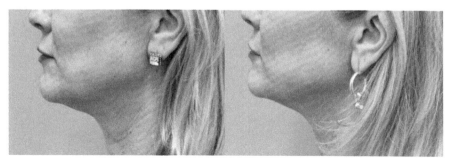

Fig. 4. A 51-year-old woman with submental and neck lift results from single treatment of Sofwave at 2 weeks follow-up. Before/after lateral images.

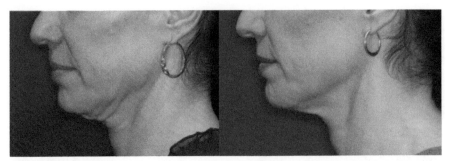

Fig. 5. A 54-year-old woman with submental lift results from single treatment of Ulthera at 3 months follow-up. Before and after lateral images. (*Courtesy of* Dr Jennifer Levine, New York, NY.)

with MFUS. Posttreatment adverse effects include edema, erythema, ecchymosis, transient facial asymmetry, and post-inflammatory pigmentation and are self-liming in nature.[4,14,22,23] In a review of 307 patients who underwent facial MFUS treatments, the most commonly reported events were transient erythema and edema posttreatment.[22] Other events include wheals or striations likely secondary to inadequate coupling of the transducer to the skin.[22] Rare events include post-inflammatory hyperpigmentation due to the use of the 4.5 mm transducer where there was insufficient tissue depth ($n = 2$) and paresis ($n = 1$).[22] In a single-center study in Paris, France, all 233 patients experienced temporary (<1 hour) erythema posttreatment, and 7 patients had continued erythema 12 to 24 hours posttreatment. In the same cohort, six patients had edema lasting 3 days, eight experienced continued pain that did not interfere with social activities, and six experienced transient numbness.[22]

CONTRAINDICATIONS AND LIMITATIONS

MFUS is a well-tolerated procedure; few contraindications have been documented in literature.[24] Absolute contraindications include infection or open skin lesions at the proposed treatment areas, active severe or cystic acne, electric implants, or metallic implants. Relative contraindications include treatment directly over keloid, implants, dermal fillers, or patient health indications that would impair healing and smoking.[11,25]

MFUS and IUB are limited to patients with mild to moderate skin sagging and wrinkling. Those with severe sagging and wrinkling would more likely benefit from surgical face-lift procedures.[21,26] Patients with severe sagging were more likely to be nonresponders to MFUS.[26] In addition, MFUS was less likely to be successful in patients with BMI higher than 30 as demonstrated by Oni and colleagues, in which no change was detected in 54.5% of patients whose BMI exceeded 30 kg/m^2 or in 12.2% of patients whose BMI was $\leq$30 kg/m^2.[11]

RESULTS IN LITERATURE

The efficacy of MFUS has been well-documented and demonstrated in clinical practice. Kerscher and colleagues demonstrated that at day 3 posttreatment, skin temperature remained in the physiologic range, with stable transepidermal water loss, hydration, and erythema.[24] Suh and colleagues in a cohort of 11 patients assessed histologic changes after one-single treatment. Based on the skin biopsy of these 11 patients, 2 months after treatment, they found that skin after treatment greater dermal collagen with thickening of

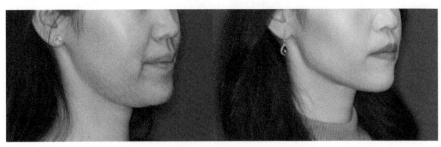

Fig. 6. A 30-year-old woman with submental lift results from single treatment of Ulthera at 3 months follow-up. Before and after lateral images. (*Courtesy of* Dr Jennifer Levine, New York, NY.)

the dermis and straightening of elastic fibers in the reticular dermis.[4]

Clinically, Suh and colleagues found that in 22 patients, 77% reported much improvement of nasolabial folds.[4] Oni and colleagues demonstrated in 93 patients in a blind reviewer study that there was observed improvement in skin laxity in 58.1% of patients. In those patients, at day 90, 65.6% of patients perceived improvement in the skin laxity of the lower half of their face/neck.[11] In a 36-subject blind rater prospective cohort study, Alam and colleagues demonstrated that there was clinically significant brow lift, with a mean elevation in eyebrow height of 1.7 mm ($P = .00001$) at 90 days after treatment.[27] Lee and colleagues in 10 patients demonstrated that two treatment passes with a 4-MHz, 4.5-mm probe was used first, followed by the 7-MHz, 3.0-mm probe yielded 80% clinical improvement 90 days after treatment based on two blinded clinician assessments and 90% subjective improvement.[18]

Subjectively, patients report high satisfaction with treatment results. Montes and colleagues in a survey of 52 patients who underwent lower face and submental MFUS demonstrated that half of patients undergoing MFU-V were Very Satisfied or Satisfied with their results and a large number reported their treatment outcome met or exceeded their expectations. Fifty percent believed they looked 1 to 15 years younger and 73% would recommend the treatment to others.[28]

A multicenter study of 58 subjects treated with IUB technology on the face and neck found an improvement of 1 to 3 Elastosis Score units in 86% of subjects using the Fitzpatrick Wrinkle and Elastosis Scale for perioral and periorbital regions. Surveys also demonstrated that 72% noted improvement in wrinkle appearance. No device-related adverse events were reported.[15,16] Examples of clinical results with Sofwave for eyebrow lift (**Fig. 3**) and submental lift (**Fig. 4**) are shown. Examples of clinical results with Ulthera for submental lift (**Figs. 5** and **6**) are shown.

SUMMARY

Ultrasound energy can be delivered to the dermal tissues, while sparing the epidermis, to induce thermal injury and subsequent collagen remodeling, leading to a lifting and tightening effect of the skin. The results are apparent, consistent, and reproducible with significant changes both at the histologic and clinical level. Boasting high patient satisfaction rates, minimal recovery time, and an excellent safety profile, ultrasound modalities serve as an attractive option for patients with mild to moderate laxity of the skin looking for noninvasive facial rejuvenation in the eyebrow, submentum, and/or neck region. As a relatively newer modality with ongoing research, ultrasound technology is an effective, nonsurgical option for facial rejuvenation available in our armamentarium that will continue to evolve and expand in its clinical applications.

CLINICS CARE POINTS

- The ideal candidate for ultrasound therapy for facial rejuvenation is patients who have mild to moderate laxity of the skin on the face and desire a nonsurgical "lifting" effect of the eyebrow, submentum, and/or neck.
- Careful patient selection and management of expectations are essential to achieving a satisfied patient.
- Because ultrasound is not chromophore-dependent, it is safe for all Fitzpatrick skin types.
- The Ulthera system can target various tissue depths between 1.5 and 4.5 mm and uses in-unit ultrasound imaging to verify targeted tissue depth and underlying structures, whereas the Sofwave system targets the mid-dermis up to 2 mm with no need for ultrasound imaging.
- Both the Ulthera and Sofwave systems require two passes for each treatment, with the exception of treatment of thinner-skinned periorbital area, which only require one pass with the Ulthera system.
- Pain associated with the treatment is well tolerated and patients do well with a combination of topical anesthetics and oral NSAID.

DISCLOSURE

Dr J.D. Bloom is a consultant, advisory board member, speaker's bureau member, trainer and clinical investigator for Galderma and Allergan. He is also a consultant, advisory board member, speaker's bureau member and trainer for Revance Aesthetics. Dr A. Wong and Dr A.S. Lowery have no disclosures.

REFERENCES

1. Brobst RW, Ferguson M, Perkins SW. Ulthera: Initial and Six Month Results. Facial Plast Surg Clin North Am 2012;20(2):163–76.
2. Gliklich RE, White WM, Slayton MH, et al. Clinical Pilot Study of Intense Ultrasound Therapy to Deep

Dermal Facial Skin and Subcutaneous Tissues. Arch Facial Plast Surg 2007;9(2):88–95.

3. Brobst RW, Ferguson M, Perkins SW. Noninvasive treatment of the neck. Facial Plast Surg Clin North Am 2014;22(2):191–202.

4. Suh DH, Shin MK, Lee SJ. Intense focused ultrasound tightening in Asian skin: clinical and pathologic results. Dermatol Surg 2011;37(11):1595–602.

5. Aşiran Serdar Z, Aktaş Karabay E, Tatlıparmak A, et al. Efficacy of high-intensity focused ultrasound in facial and neck rejuvenation. J Cosmet Dermatol 2020;19(2):353–8.

6. Wulkan AJ, Fabi SG, Green JB. Microfocused Ultrasound for Facial Photorejuvenation: A Review. Facial Plast Surg 2016;32(03):269–75.

7. Minkis K, Alam M. Ultrasound Skin Tightening. Dermatol Clin 2014;32(1):71–7.

8. Gutowski KA. Microfocused Ultrasound for Skin Tightening. Clin Plast Surg 2016;43(3):577–82.

9. Bader KB, Makin IRS, Abramowicz JS. Ultrasound for Aesthetic Applications: A Review of Biophysical Mechanisms and Safety. J Ultrasound Med 2022; 41(7):1597–607.

10. Pak CS, Lee YK, Jeong JH, et al. Safety and efficacy of Ulthera in the rejuvenation of aging lower eyelids: a pivotal clinical trial. Aesthetic Plast Surg 2014; 38(5):861–8.

11. Oni G, Hoxworth R, Teotia S, et al. Evaluation of a Microfocused Ultrasound System for Improving Skin Laxity and Tightening in the Lower Face. Aesthetic Surg J 2014;34(7):1099–110.

12. Laubach HJ, Makin IR, Barthe PG, et al. Intense focused ultrasound: evaluation of a new treatment modality for precise microcoagulation within the skin. Dermatol Surg 2008;34(5):727–34.

13. White WM, Makin IRS, Barthe PG, et al. Selective Creation of Thermal Injury Zones in the Superficial Musculoaponeurotic System Using Intense Ultrasound Therapy. Arch Facial Plast Surg 2007;9(1): 22–9.

14. Chan NPY, Shek SYN, Yu CS, et al. Safety study of transcutaneous focused ultrasound for noninvasive skin tightening in Asians. Laser Surg Med 2011;43(5):366–75.

15. Wang JV. The use of ultrasound in aesthetics: review and update. San Clemente, CA: Sofwave, Inc.; 2020.

16. Amir R. A novel approach to treating wrinkles and laxity of the face and neck using Intense Ultrasound Beam. 2020. Available at: https://sofwave.com/physicians/technology/. Accessed January 3, 2023.

17. Ulthera Update White Paper: Introduction of the 1.5 mm Shallow Transducer. Available at: https://www.casas.md/files/2015/12/15mm-transducer-white-paper-1000674b.pdf. Acessed January 3, 2023.

18. Lee HS, Jang WS, Cha Y-J, et al. Multiple Pass Ultrasound Tightening of Skin Laxity of the Lower Face and Neck. Dermatol Surg 2012;38(1):20–7.

19. Sasaki GH, Tevez A. Clinical efficacy and safety of focused-image ultrasonography: a 2-year experience. Aesthet Surg J 2012;32(5):601–12.

20. Fabi SG. Noninvasive skin tightening: focus on new ultrasound techniques. Clin Cosmet Investig Dermatol 2015;8:47–52.

21. Shome D, Vadera S, Ram MS, et al. Use of Microfocused Ultrasound for Skin Tightening of Mid and Lower Face. Plast Reconstr Surg Glob Open 2019; 7(12):e2498.

22. Hitchcock TM, Dobke MK. Review of the safety profile for microfocused ultrasound with visualization. J Cosmet Dermatol 2014;13(4):329–35.

23. Fabi SG. Microfocused ultrasound with visualization for skin tightening and lifting: my experience and a review of the literature. Dermatol Surg 2014; 40(Suppl 12):S164–7.

24. Kerscher M, Nurrisyanti AT, Eiben-Nielson C, et al. Skin physiology and safety of microfocused ultrasound with visualization for improving skin laxity. Clin Cosmet Investig Dermatol 2019;12:71–9.

25. MacGregor JL, Tanzi EL. Microfocused ultrasound for skin tightening. Semin Cutan Med Surg 2013; 32(1):18–25.

26. Friedman O, Isman G, Koren A, et al. Intense focused ultrasound for neck and lower face skin tightening a prospective study. J Cosmet Dermatol 2020;19(4):850–4.

27. Alam M, White LE, Martin N, et al. Ultrasound tightening of facial and neck skin: a rater-blinded prospective cohort study. J Am Acad Dermatol 2010; 62(2):262–9.

28. Montes JR, Santos E. Patient Satisfaction Following Treatment With Microfocused Ultrasound With Visualization: Results of a Retrospective Cross-Sectional Survey. J Drugs Dermatol 2019;18(1): 75–9.

Neuromodulators for Skin

Anya Costeloe, DO[a,b,c,*], Angela Nguyen, BS[a], Corey Maas, MD[a,b]

KEYWORDS

- Neurotoxins • Botulinum toxin • Microtox • OnabotulinumtoxinA • AbobotulinumtoxinA
- IncobotulinumtoxinA • DaxibotulinumtoxinA

KEY POINTS

- Injection of botulinum toxin type A (BoNTA) in the dermal and subdermal layers can lead to various physiologic changes in the skin including reduced sebum production and smoothing of the skin caused by minimizing the tethering effects of muscles attached to the skin.
- The optimal BoNTA dose and concentration may vary in different areas of the face and neck based on the interaction between the skin and muscle, the skin thickness, and tissue strength in the area.
- Clinical outcomes of BoNTA treatment depend on the skills and training of the injector; however, the properties of the toxin used, its concentration, and the total volume injected are also critical factors.
- Neurotoxins are generally safe; however, side effects are possible and new data are emerging on the long-term use of BoNTA and atrophy of target muscles.

HISTORY AND CURRENT PRACTICE CONDITIONS

The contemporary applications of botulinum toxin have changed dramatically over the past 10 years. The first two decades of use of toxins were hallmarked by the presence of only one US first-in-class product; trepidation among European aesthetic thought leaders and providers; and advances in dose, technique, and vast expansion of applications driven by a handful of clinicians. By this decade there are five approved botulinum toxin type A (BoNTA) neuromodulators available for cosmetic use with various described indications in a multibillion dollar market that is worldwide in scope with newer products on the horizon. This decade has also demonstrated through the Food and Drug Administration (FDA) and non-FDA clinical trials that the full potential of this class of pharmacologic agents is only now being reached. Practiced dosage norms and publications assumed a false premise, without substantive data, that maximum duration of effectiveness was at approximately 3 months (the time at which less than 50% of clinical responders returned to conditions requiring retreatment).[1,2] In practice, these "intermediate" doses show a response as it relates to duration following a bell curve subject to proper delivery to the target site and variation in response by individuals.[2] Escalating dose studies have given good evidence of this variation, whereas higher doses are safely administered in higher concentrations (less diluent), which move the median effective duration consistently beyond 6 months with some responders showing much longer duration of effect.[3–6]

These newer findings and possible movement of higher dosing norms may prove to catch up with what is already proven as the desirable clinical interval of approximately 6 months as evidenced by annual average patient-driven treatment frequency of 1.9 treatments per year. In short, irrespective of the frown, wrinkle, or line severity, patients return for retreatment on average every 6 months and it has been demonstrated that patients are satisfied with two treatments a year.[7] It will be interesting to see as the clinical dosing norms increase if retreatment frequency changes or stays at an average of 1.9 treatments per year.

The use of BoNTA continues to rise and it was the most popular nonsurgical cosmetic procedure

[a] Facial Plastic and Reconstructive Surgery, The Maas Clinic, 2400 Clay Street, San Francisco, CA 94115, USA; [b] California Pacific Heights Medical Center, San Francisco, CA, USA; [c] Premier Plastic Surgery, Palo Alto, CA, USA
* Corresponding author. 2400 Clay street, San Francisco, CA 94115.
E-mail address: anyacosteloe@gmail.com

Facial Plast Surg Clin N Am 31 (2023) 511–519
https://doi.org/10.1016/j.fsc.2023.06.002
1064-7406/23/© 2023 Elsevier Inc. All rights reserved.

in 2020 in every age group with 4.4 million people in the United States receiving treatment.[8] As these safe and effective products move from the hands of well-trained aesthetic core physicians to nurses and other physician extenders and general acceptance of these pharmacologic agents as low risk and routine aesthetic skin treatments increases, more patients are being well-served with an ongoing need for educational opportunity for mid-level providers.

CURRENT BOTULINUM TOXIN TYPE A AGENTS, DILUTIONS, AND CONCENTRATIONS

The clinically available products in current use have doubled in the last decade with multiple serotype A toxins on the market. In 2010, the FDA first approved the 150-kDa molecule incobotulinum-toxinA for the treatment of cervical dystonia in adults and blepharospasm in patients previously treated with onabotulinumtoxinA (Xeomin, Merz Pharmaceuticals, LLC, Frankfurt, Germany), and in 2011 it was approved for cosmetic use. Xeomin was stripped of accompanying proteins and adver-tised as the pure, additive-free toxin with the major advantage being that unopened vials can be stored at room temperature. In 2019, the FDA approved prabotulinumtoxinA (Jeuveau, Evolus Pharma, Santa Barbara, CA) for the temporary improvement in the appearance of moderate to severe glabellar lines associated with corrugator and/or procerus muscle activity in adult patients. Most recently, daxibotulinumtoxinA (DAXXIFY; Revance Thera-peutics, Inc, Newark, CA) was approved for the temporary treatment of moderate to severe glabellar rhytids. Thus, five BoNTA products repre-sent the current palette of available serotype A neu-romodulators: Botox, Dysport, Xeomin, Jeuveau, and DAXXIFY are summarized in **Table 1**.

DAXXIFY (DAXI) was approved by the FDA in 2022 as an injectable for treating glabellar rhytids but it was originally formulated as a topical gel with the excipient protein intended to assist in moving the toxin across the epithelial barrier.[9,10] However, although the study results demonstrated only a one- or two-point or greater improvement in the lateral canthal lines baseline severity at 8 weeks with statistically significant results compared with the placebo in a small study popu-lation and was well tolerated, the study was ulti-mately discontinued in favor of developing the injectable DAXI.

DAXI consists of 150-kDa purified daxibotuli-numtoxinA (RTT150, a 150-kDa BoNTA) and a 35–amino acid highly positively charged peptide (RTP004) that forms a strong electrostatic bond with the toxin referred to as peptide exchange

technology, and a surfactant (polysorbate 20), buffers, and a sugar that protects the neurotoxin during the drying process.[11–13] The stabilizing peptide and the polysorbate-20 promote thermal stability of the toxin and permits the lyophilized form to be stable at room temperature for up to 3 years before reconstitution.[11] The advertised advantage of DAXI is the increased duration of ef-ficacy with clinical trial data demonstrating a 24-week median duration of effect (defined as time over which none or mild glabellar line severity score was maintained) and a 27.1-week median time to return to baseline.[12,13] The researchers attribute this to the proprietary peptide exchange technology that DAXI is formulated with; however, studies have found that other BoNTA products injected at higher doses have a similar prolonged duration of effect.[3–6] The DAXI toxin and its increased duration of efficacy raises the inter-esting question regarding dosing of the existing toxins on the market and whether higher doses of these toxins would similarly result in prolonged efficacy. The senior author's (C.S.M.) 2021 clinical trial data demonstrated that when treating the glabella with higher doses of incobotulinumtoxinA, there was a dose-dependent increase in duration of efficacy. The median duration of effect was 120 days with 20 U, 180 days with 60 U, and 270 days with 100 U.[4] The 6-month results for the group receiving 60 U are shown in **Fig. 1**. Further large-scale studies are needed to define the upper limits of safe duration of effect while providing clinically beneficial results as it relates to skin and facial expression.

Although there are five BoNTA products currently available, emerging neuromodulators continue to be developed and tested in clinical trials. A second liquid formulation of abobotuli-numtoxinA, compared with the FDA-approved ready-to-use serotype B Myobloc, is currently un-der FDA consideration.[14] A new serotype E prod-uct is also under consideration by the FDA, which showed an onset within 24 hours and dura-tion of effect between 14 and 30 days at the high-est dose in phase II clinical trials.[15] The study results support its development for therapeutic or cosmetic applications where a faster onset of ac-tion and shorter duration of effect are preferable.

Reconstitution

The preparation of BoNTA for injection involves reconstituting the toxin powder with a diluent solu-tion. The manufacturer-recommended diluent for each of the five toxins approved for cosmetic use is unpreserved saline (0.9% sodium chloride injec-tion USP)[16–20]; however, many practitioners prefer

Table 1
Current FDA-approved BoNTA products on the market

	OnaBTXA	AboBTXA	IncoBTXA	praBTXA	DaxiBTXA
Brand name	Botox	Dysport	Xeomin	Jeuveau	Daxxify
Company	Allergan, Inc	Galderma	Merz Aesthetics	Evolus Pharma	Revance
Cosmetic use approval year	2002	2009	2010	2019	2022
Approved cosmetic indications	Glabellar lines Lateral canthal lines Forehead lines	Glabellar lines in patients <65 y	Glabellar lines	Glabellar lines	Glabellar lines
Glabellar line treatment dose	20 U	50 U	20 U	20 U	40 U
Size	900 kDa	500 kDa	150 kDa	900 kDa	150 kDa
Active substance	Botulinum toxin A complex	Botulinum toxin A complex	Botulinum toxin A	Botulinum toxin A	Botulinum toxin and stabilizing protein
Excipients	Sodium chloride, 500 μg HSA	Lactose, 125 μg HSA	Sucrose, 1 mg HSA	Sodium chloride, HSA	PS20, sugar, buffer, excipient peptide (RTP004)
Units per vial	50 or 100	300 or 500	50 or 100	100	100
Diluent (mL)	2.5	1.5 or 2.5	2.5	2.5	1.2
Concentration	4 U/0.1 mL	10 U/0.05 mL or 10 U/0.08 mL	4 U/0.1 mL	4 U/0.1 mL	8 U/0.1 mL
Storage unopened vial	Refrigerate	Refrigerate	Room temp or refrigerate	Refrigerate	Room temp or refrigerate
Storage life after reconstitution (h)	24	24	24	24	72

Abbreviations: AboBTXA, abobotulinumtoxinA; DaxiBTXA, daxibotulinumtoxinA; HSA, human serum albumin; IncoBTXA, incobotulinumtoxinA; OnaBTXA, onabotulinumtoxinA.

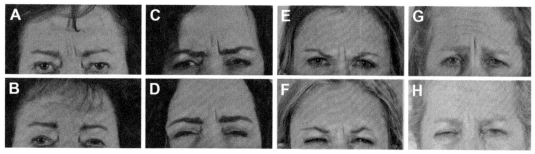

Fig. 1. Before and after photographs of patients at baseline (*A, C, E, G*) and 6 months after (*B, D, F, H*) treating the glabellar area with 60 U of incobotulinumtoxinA.

preserved saline because it minimizes pain with injection and it has been shown that it does not affect the potency of Botox.[21,22] The diluent and storage recommendations for each commercially available toxin are summarized in **Table 1**.

Concentration

The amount of diluent used to reconstitute BoNTA can affect treatment outcomes in several ways because it determines the concentration of toxin in the final solution. The choice of concentration depends on the target muscle and the desired effect. For onabotulinumtoxinA, this is typically between 1 and 4 mL of saline or bacteriostatic water.[17] The commonly used concentrations may elevate as average dosing rises based on studies showing longer duration of effectiveness with higher doses.[3–6]

The amount of diluent also affects the diffusion and spread of the toxin after injection. More diluent may promote wider distribution, potentially affecting adjacent muscles and increasing the risk of unwanted effects. Less diluent can lead to a more localized effect and the overall volume can influence the precision of injection. Smaller amounts of diluent may make it easier to deliver the toxin precisely into the target muscle, whereas larger amounts may make it more challenging to control the injection site. Diluent volume also affects the calculation of the final dosage to be administered and proper dosage calculation is crucial to ensure the desired therapeutic effect while minimizing the risk of adverse events.

Physiologic Impacts on the Skin Architecture

When applied consistently to the mimetic muscles, botulinum neuromodulators are impactful and repeated treatments with BoNTA can lead to several changes in the architecture of the skin. The primary effect of BoNTA is the temporary relaxation of targeted muscles, which reduces the appearance of wrinkles and lines on the skin's surface. Muscle relaxation depends on the administered dose and on the capacity of the terminal axon to regenerate.[23] Over time, this repeated muscle relaxation can lead to secondary changes in the skin. To understand these changes, it is important to understand the relationship between skin and facial muscles, which is influenced by skin thickness, dermal muscle insertion, and strength of connective tissue between the muscle and the skin.[24,25]

One significant change in the architecture of the skin is the reduction in dynamic wrinkles caused by repetitive muscle contractions. The repeated injection of BoNTA prevents these muscle contractions, allowing the skin to smooth out and diminish the appearance of wrinkles associated with facial expressions. Additionally, the use of BoNTA can result in improved skin texture and quality. The relaxation of muscles can lead to a decrease in excessive muscle movements, which may contribute to the prevention of deeper lines and creases from forming. This effect can provide the skin with a more youthful and refreshed appearance.

However, BoNTA treatments primarily address dynamic wrinkles caused by muscle movement and do not directly affect other skin components, such as collagen or elastin. Consequently, the long-term effects of BoNTA on skin architecture beyond the reduction of muscle-related wrinkles may vary and depend on individual factors, such as age, skin condition, and treatment frequency.

Physiologic Skin Changes with Repeated Treatments and Further Applications

Injection of BoNTA in the dermal and subdermal layers can lead to various physiologic changes in the skin including reduced sebum production and smoothing of the skin caused by minimizing the tethering effects of muscles attached to the skin. BoNTA's effect on sebum production has been studied for the last decade with multiple studies showing promising results.[26–28] In multiple studies it was demonstrated that the delivery of small aliquots of dilute BoNTA in the dermal or subdermal plane decreases sebum production by the sebaceous glands,[26,29] and the term "microtox" was coined. This application on BoNTA is beneficial for individuals with oily or acne-prone skin as demonstrated in preliminary studies, because it may help to control excessive oiliness and minimize the occurrence of breakouts.[26,30] The superficial injection of BoNTA allows for patients to maintain muscle movement allowing for a more natural and less "frozen" result. Further studies have combined BoNTA with hyaluronic acid in a microtox and micro–hyaluronic acid formulation to enhance skin hydration.[31] Theoretically, the relaxation of muscles can help minimize transepidermal water loss, allowing the skin to retain moisture more effectively. This can contribute to a plumper, more hydrated appearance.

The muscle relaxation induced by BoNTA injections can improve blood circulation in the treated areas. A recent meta-analysis of studies done in animal models showed that BoNT A and B serotypes cause vasodilation; it increased vessel diameter in arteries by 40% and in veins by 46% and reduced thrombosis by 85% in arteries and 79% in veins compared with saline controls.[32] They also found that BoNT increased flap survival by 26%. Further studies are warranted in humans and if similar improvement of blood flow is demonstrated, it will have valuable aesthetic applications. Enhanced blood flow brings more oxygen and nutrients to the skin, promoting a healthier complexion and supporting the skin's natural repair processes.

Another area of ongoing research is the use of BoNTA to treat rosacea and facial flushing associated with menopause.[33] It is thought that BoNTA may improve flushing by its ability to suppress acetylcholine release in the cutaneous vasodilatory system and by inhibiting inflammatory mediators, such as calcitonin gene-related peptide and substance P.[34] However, there are conflicting data on the efficacy of BoNTA in treating these disorders and further studies are warranted.[35]

Multiple studies have demonstrated that BoNTA improves the appearance of facial and neck scars by relieving muscle tension from the scar as it heals and through BoNTA's anti-inflammatory properties. A study looking at 15 thyroidectomy patients showed that patients who had 20 to 65 U of BoNTA injected into the scar within 10 days of surgery had superior scar scores and patient satisfaction compared with patients receiving saline injections.[36] Three clinical studies have investigated the use of BoNTA to improve scar appearance. All three studies administered intralesional BoNTA at 2.5 U/cm^3 once a month for a total of 3 months and found that patients receiving BoNTA had improvement in satisfaction, erythema, and itching.[37–39] It is worth noting that although these physiologic changes can occur as a result of BoNTA treatments, their extent and duration may vary among individuals. Such factors as treatment frequency, dosage, and individual skin characteristics can influence the specific effects experienced by each person.

Treatment Recommendations by Anatomic Region

Off-label uses of BoNTA include treatment of horizontal forehead lines, horizontal nasal lines ("bunny lines"), ptotic brow, nasal tip ptosis, excessive nasal flaring, excessive gingival show with smiling ("gummy smile"), long upper lip ("lip flip"), downturned smile, perioral lines, masseter hypertrophy, dimpled chin, and platysmal bands of the neck. The injection sites and doses typically injected by the authors of each type of BoNTA are summarized in **Fig. 2** and **Table 2**.

Complications and Management

Botulinum toxin treatments for the face and neck have been generally well-tolerated, but like any

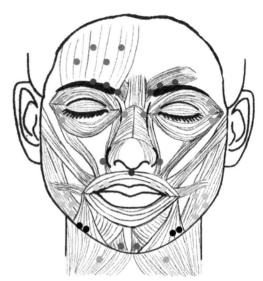

Fig. 2. Face and neck injection site. *Colored circles* represent sites of BoNTA injection. Units of BoNTA per target muscles are summarized in **Table 2**.

medical procedure, they can have complications and side effects. The most common reported side effects associated with BoNTA treatments are injection site side effects including bruising and swelling and headache and muscle asymmetry.[40] More serious side effects are possible yet rare. Systemic effects could include muscle weakness, swallowing difficulties, or respiratory problems if BoNTA is absorbed into the bloodstream.[41] Although extremely rare, there is a theoretical risk of allergic reactions to BoNTA and several cases have been reported in the literature.[42]

In the upper face, the more common complications are eyelid and eyebrow ptosis. A rarer complication is periocular edema, which has been attributed to retention of lymphatic fluid in the infraorbital region. It is hypothesized that there is a disruption of lymphatic outflow because of weakening of the orbicularis oculi and its sphincteric pumping function.[43]

In the lower face, potential complications include oral motor insufficiency, decreased dental show with smiling, and asymmetrical smile. Specific complications that can occur when targeting the platysma include dysphagia, neck weakness, and dry mouth.[44] Treating masseter hypertrophy with BoNTA can result in smile and facial asymmetry and weakness in chewing.[40]

If excessive muscle weakness is observed, it may be necessary to administer an antidote or reversal agent, such as an acetylcholinesterase inhibitor, to counteract the effects of the toxin. These medications can help restore muscle

Table 2
Total units of each BoNTA injected in different muscle groups in the face and neck (units are equally distributed between 2 sides where relevant)

Color[a]	Treatment Area	Targeted Muscles	OnaBTXA	AboBTXA	IncoBTXA	praBTXA	DaxiBTXA[b]
Dark blue	Vertical glabellar lines	Corrugator	10–25	60	10–25	10–25	40
Grey	Forehead lines	Frontalis	5–10	15–30	5–10	5–10	—
Medium blue	Smile lines	Orbicularis oculi	10–20	30–60	10–20	10–20	—
Light blue	Brow elevation	Superolateral orbicularis oculi	3–5	9–15	3–5	3–5	—
Light green	Horizontal glabellar lines	Procerus	3–10	9–30	3–10	3–10	—
Dark green	Bunny lines	Nasalis	5	15	5	5	—
Maroon	Nasal tip ptosis	Depressor septi	5–8	15–21	5–8	5–8	—
Red	Gummy smile	Levator labii superioris alaeque nasi	4	12	4	4	—
Yellow	Lip flip	Orbicularis oculi	4	12	4	4	—
Black	Marionette lines	Depressor anguli oris	5–10	15–30	5–10	5–10	—
Purple	Dimpled chin	Mentalis	5	15	5	5	—
Pink	Masseter hypertrophy	Masseter	20–40	60–120	20–40	20–40	—
Orange	Neck bands	Platysma	10 (per band)	30 (per band)	10 (per band)	10 (per band)	—

Abbreviations: AboBTXA, abobotulinumtoxinA; DaxiBTXA, daxibotulinumtoxinA; IncoBTXA, incobotulinumtoxinA. OnaBTXA, onabotulinumtoxinA; PraBTXA, pravobotulinumtoxinA.
[a] Color refers to injection sites illustrated in **Fig. 1**.
[b] Data only available for treatment of glabellar rhytids.

function and reduce the duration of the adverse effects. Asymmetry or unintended muscle paralysis can often be addressed by carefully administering additional injections to rebalance the muscle activity. This may involve injecting the antagonist muscles to counteract the effects of the toxin and restore a more natural appearance.

Studies are currently being conducted on the long-term effects of BoNTA use as more data become available on patients using Botox for several decades. One area of research is the short- and long-term effects of BoNTA injection on muscle mass and fibers. Fibrosis of muscle fibers and muscle atrophy with necrosis after BoNTA injection have been reported in several studies. A systematic review looked at the relationship between BoNTA injections and muscle atrophy and found that there was reduction of muscle base ranging from 18% to 60% after one to multiple BoNTA injections in human and animal models.[45] Furthermore, there was no complete muscle recovery in the six human studies included in the review. Borodic and Ferrante[46] showed a morphometric reduction in orbicularis muscle fibers at 3 months after BoNTA injections, whereas another study showed a 19.6% reduction in the diameter of vastus lateralis muscle fibers 2 to 4 years after BoNTA injections.[47] These findings indicate that BoNTA injections may result in long-term muscle atrophy and current studies are looking at how this may impact the bony skeleton and potential bone loss.[48]

NEUROTOXIN USE IN FACIAL PARALYSIS

The most common targets for chemodenervation for patients with facial nerve synkinesis are the ipsilateral orbicularis oculi, mentalis, depressor anguli oris (DAO), buccinator, corrugator muscles, and the ipsilateral and/or contralateral frontalis, depending on the patient synkinesis pattern. For selective patients, the contralateral depressor labii inferioris is targeted to achieve lower lip symmetry during a smile. Overactivated orbicularis oris and DAO is frequently encountered in patients with synkinesis within the lower third of the face and presents as incomplete oral commissure excursion and raised lower lip height ipsilaterally. The ipsilateral DAO and orbicularis oris are targeted to increase commissure elevation with less orbicularis contraction. In some patients, the contralateral depressor labii inferioris is targeted to elevate the contralateral lower lip to achieve better symmetry.[49]

Botulinum toxins can also be used to predict surgical outcomes in facial nerve paralysis patients. A prospective analysis of 23 patients undergoing DAO muscle block followed by resection for nonflaccid paralysis discovered that the nerve block was useful in predicting oral commissure excursion symmetry in response to resection; however, commissure symmetry was significantly better following resection versus the block.[50] Additionally, neuromodulators can help with functional deficits in patients experiencing facial nerve paralysis. Longino and colleagues[51] performed a retrospective review analyzing 29 patients with synkinesis, jaw tightness, pain, and swallowing discomfort. The patients underwent chemodenervation of the posterior belly of the digastric, performed under electromyographic direction, and had significant improvement of jaw tightness and swallowing without reported adverse effects.

BOTULINUM TOXINS AND THE FUTURE

The future of botulinum toxins in aesthetic treatments of the skin, face, neck, and other areas is expected to continue evolving and expanding. Predicted trends and advancements include improved formulations, combination therapies, personalized treatments, expanded treatment areas, and longer lasting effects. Ongoing research and development efforts are focused on refining botulinum toxin formulations to enhance their effectiveness, duration, and precision. This includes the exploration of new types of botulinum toxins with different properties and characteristics. Researchers are investigating ways to prolong the duration of botulinum toxin effects by exploring novel formulations, delivery techniques, and adjunct therapies that can extend the longevity of results and reduce the frequency of treatments. Combination therapies with other aesthetic procedures, such as dermal fillers or laser treatments, to achieve more comprehensive and synergistic results are on the rise.[52] This trend is likely to continue as practitioners explore combination therapies tailored to individual patient needs.

The future of aesthetic medicine aims to provide more personalized treatments. Advancements in technology, such as imaging and three-dimensional modeling, may enable practitioners to create customized treatment plans that consider an individual's unique facial anatomy, skin condition, and treatment goals. Aesthetic trends are also shifting toward more natural-looking results, where facial expressions are preserved while achieving subtle rejuvenation. Future developments in botulinum toxin treatments may prioritize achieving these natural and harmonious outcomes.

SUMMARY

BoNTA is a potent neurotoxin that has various aesthetic and functional applications not only in the face and neck but in the entire body and is being used to treat muscle, skin, and other target organs. An important area of for future research is optimizing dosing and concentration as it relates to duration, which varies based on the anatomic and functional targets.

CLINICS CARE POINTS

- Neuromodulators have been shown to decrease sebum production and this finding is important for treating patients with hyperhidrosis and acne.
- There have been studies looking at the effect of BoNTA on vasculature, scars, rosacea, and facial flushing and there are some promising data; however, larger scale studies are needed for conclusive data.

REFERENCES

1. Flynn TC. Botulinum toxin: examining duration of effect in facial aesthetic applications. Am J Clin Dermatol 2010;11(3):183–99.
2. Carruthers JA, Lowe NJ, Menter MA, et al. A multicenter, double-blind, randomized, placebo-controlled study of the efficacy and safety of

botulinum toxin type A in the treatment of glabellar lines. J Am Acad Dermatol 2002;46(6):840–9.

3. Kerscher M, Fabi S, Fischer T, et al. IncobotulinumtoxinA demonstrates safety and prolonged duration of effect in a dose-ranging study for glabellar lines. J Drugs Dermatol 2020;19(10):985–91.

4. Polacco MA, Singleton AE, Barnes CH, et al. A double-blind, randomized clinical trial to determine effects of increasing doses and dose-response relationship of incobotulinumtoxinA in the treatment of glabellar rhytids. Aesthetic Surg J 2021;41(6):NP500–11.

5. Joseph J, Moradi A, Lorenc ZP, et al. AbobotulinumtoxinA for the treatment of moderate-to-severe glabellar lines: a randomized, dose-escalating, double-blind study. J Drugs Dermatol 2021;20(9):980–7.

6. Joseph JH, Maas C, Palm MD, et al. Safety, pharmacodynamic response, and treatment satisfaction with onabotulinumtoxinA 40 U, 60 U, and 80 U in subjects with moderate to severe dynamic glabellar lines. Aesthetic Surg J 2022;42(11):1318–27.

7. Schlessinger J, Cohen JL, Shamban A, et al. A multicenter study to evaluate subject satisfaction with two treatments of abobotulinumtoxinA a year in the glabellar lines. Dermatol Surg 2021;47(4):504–9.

8. American Society of Plastic Surgeons InternetNational Clearinghouse of Plastic Surgery Procedural Statistics (2020) Available at: https://www.plasticsurgery.org/documents/News/Statistics/2020/plastic-surgery-statistics-full-report-2020.pdf. Accessed May 26, 2023.

9. Brandt F, O'Connell C, Cazzaniga A, et al. Efficacy and safety evaluation of a novel botulinum toxin topical gel for the treatment of moderate to severe lateral canthal lines. Dermatol Surg 2010;36(Suppl 4):2111–8.

10. Glogau R, Blitzer A, Brandt F, et al. Results of a randomized, double-blind, placebo-controlled study to evaluate the efficacy and safety of a botulinum toxin type A topical gel for the treatment of moderate-to-severe lateral canthal lines. J Drugs Dermatol 2012;11(1):38–45.

11. Malmirchegini R, Too P, Oliyai C, Joshi A. Revance's novel peptide excipient, RTP004, and its role in stabilizing daxibotulinumtoxinA (DAXI) against aggregation. Poster presented at: TOXINS 2019; January 16–19, 2019; Copenhagen, Denmark

12. Carruthers JD, Fagien S, Joseph JH, et al. DaxibotulinumtoxinA for injection for the treatment of glabellar lines: results from each of two multicenter, randomized, double-blind, placebo-controlled, phase 3 studies (SAKURA 1 and SAKURA 2). Plast Reconstr Surg 2020;145(1):45–58.

13. Bertucci V, Solish N, Kaufman-Janette J, et al. DaxibotulinumtoxinA for Injection has a prolonged duration of response in the treatment of glabellar lines: pooled data from two multicenter, randomized, double-blind, placebo-controlled, phase 3 studies (SAKURA 1 and SAKURA 2). J Am Acad Dermatol 2020;82(4):838–45.

14. Kestemont P, Hilton S, Andriopoulos B, et al. Long-term efficacy and safety of liquid abobotulinumtoxinA formulation for moderate-to-severe glabellar lines: a phase III, double-blind, randomized, placebo-controlled and open-label study. Aesthetic Surg J 2022;42(3):301–13.

15. Yoelin SG, Dhawan SS, Vitarella D, et al. Safety and efficacy of EB-001, a novel type e botulinum toxin, in subjects with glabellar frown lines: results of a phase 2, randomized, placebo-controlled, ascending-dose study. Plast Reconstr Surg 2018;142(6):847e–55e.

16. DYSPORT® (abobotulinumtoxinA) [package insert]. Wrexham, UK: Ipsen Biopharm Ltd; Rev.; 2020.

17. BOTOX® cosmetic (onabotulinumtoxinA) [package insert]. Irvine, CA: Allergan, Inc.; Rev.; 2021.

18. XEOMIN® (incobotulinumtoxinA) [package insert]. Frankfurt, DE: Merz Pharmaceuticals GmbH; Rev.; 2021.

19. JEUVEAU™ (prabotulinumtoxinA-xvfs) [package insert]. Santa Barbara, CA: Evolus, Inc.; 2019.

20. DAXXIFY™ (daxibotulinumtoxinA-lanm) [package insert]. Newark, CA: Revance Therapeutics, Inc.; 2022.

21. Kwiat DM, Bersani TA, Bersani A. Increased patient comfort utilizing botulinum toxin type A reconstituted with preserved versus nonpreserved saline. Ophthal Plast Reconstr Surg 2004;20:186–9.

22. Carruthers J, Fagien S, Matarasso SL. Consensus recommendations on the use of botulinum toxin type A in facial aesthetics. Plast Reconstr Surg 2004;11(6):2S. Suppl 4.

23. Foran PG, Davletov B, Meunier FA. Getting muscles moving again after botulinum toxin: novel therapeutic challenges. Trends Mol Med 2003;9(7):291–9.

24. Cotofana S, Mian A, Sykes JM, et al. An update on the anatomy of the forehead compartments. Plast Reconstr Surg 2017;139(4):864e–72e.

25. Sandulescu T, Franzmann M, Jast J, et al. Facial fold and crease development: a new morphological approach and classification. Clin Anat 2019;32(4):573–84.

26. Shah AR. Use of intradermal botulinum toxin to reduce sebum production and facial pore size. J Drugs Dermatol 2008;7(9):847–50.

27. Min P, Xi W, Grassetti L, et al. Sebum production alteration after botulinum toxin type A injections for the treatment of forehead rhytides: a prospective randomized double-blind dose-comparative clinical investigation. Aesthetic Surg J 2015;35(5):600–10.

28. Kesty K, Goldberg DJ. A randomized, double-blinded study evaluating the safety and efficacy of abobotulinumtoxinA injections for oily skin of the forehead: a dose-response analysis. Dermatol Surg 2021;47(1):56–60.

29. Wu WTL. Microbotox of the lower face and neck: evolution of a personal technique and its clinical effects. Plast Reconstr Surg 2015;136(5 Suppl): 92S–100S.

30. Rose AE, Goldberg DJ. Safety and efficacy of intradermal injection of botulinum toxin for the treatment of oily skin. Dermatol Surg 2013;39(3 Pt 1):443–8.

31. Kim J. Clinical effects on skin texture and hydration of the face using microbotox and microhyaluronicacid. Plast Reconstr Surg Glob Open 2018;6(11): e1935.

32. Goldberg SH, Gehrman MD, Graham JH. Botulinum toxin A and B improve perfusion, increase flap survival, cause vasodilation, and prevent thrombosis: a systematic review and meta-analysis of controlled animal studies. Hand (N Y). 2023;18(1):22–31.

33. Odo ME, Odo LM, Farias RV, et al. Botulinum toxin for the treatment of menopausal hot flushes: a pilot study. Dermatol Surg 2011;37(11):1579–83.

34. Carmichael NME, Dostrovsky JO, Charlton MP. Peptide-mediated transdermal delivery of botulinum neurotoxin type A reduces neurogenic inflammation in the skin. Pain 2010;149(2):316–24.

35. Martina E, Diotallevi F, Radi G, et al. Therapeutic use of botulinum neurotoxins in dermatology: systematic review. Toxins 2021;13(2):120.

36. Kim YS, Lee HJ, Cho SH, et al. Early postoperative treatment of thyroidectomy scars using botulinum toxin: a split-scar, double-blind randomized controlled trial. Wound Repair Regen 2014;22(5): 605–12.

37. Elshahed AR, Elmanzalawy KS, Shehata H, et al. Effect of botulinum toxin type A for treating hypertrophic scars: a split-scar, double-blind randomized controlled trial. J Cosmet Dermatol 2020;19(9): 2252–8.

38. Elhefnawy AM. Assessment of intralesional injection of botulinum toxin type A injection for hypertrophic scars. Indian J Dermatol Venereol Leprol 2016; 82(3):279–83.

39. Xiao Z, Zhang F, Cui Z. Treatment of hypertrophic scars with intralesional botulinum toxin type A injections: a preliminary report. Aesthetic Plast Surg 2009;33(3):409–12.

40. Cavallini M, Cirillo P, Fundarò SP, et al. Safety of botulinum toxin A in aesthetic treatments: a systematic review of clinical studies. Dermatol Surg 2014; 40(5):525–36.

41. Sorensen EP, Urman C. Cosmetic complications: rare and serious events following botulinum toxin and soft tissue filler administration. J Drugs Dermatol 2015;14(5):486–91.

42. Moon IJ, Chang SE, Kim SD. First case of anaphylaxis after botulinum toxin type A injection. Clin Exp Dermatol 2017;42(7):760–2.

43. Chang YS, Chang CC, Shen JH, et al. Nonallergic eyelid edema after botulinum toxin type A injection: case report and review of literature. Medicine (Baltim) 2015;94(38):e1610.

44. Obagi S, Golubets K. Mild to moderate dysphagia following very low-dose abobotulinumtoxin A for platysmal bands. J Drugs Dermatol 2017;16(9):929–30.

45. Nassif AD, Boggio RF, Espicalsky S, et al. High precision use of botulinum toxin type A (BONT-A) in aesthetics based on muscle atrophy, is muscular architecture reprogramming a possibility? A systematic review of literature on muscle atrophy after BoNT-A injections. Toxins 2022;14(2):81.

46. Borodic GE, Ferrante R. Effects of repeated botulinum toxin injections on orbicularis oculi muscle. J Clin Neuro Ophthalmol 1992;12(2):121–7.

47. Ansved T, Odergren T, Borg K. Muscle fiber atrophy in leg muscles after botulinum toxin type A treatment of cervical dystonia. Neurology 1997;48(5):1440–2.

48. Aziz J, Awal D, Ayliffe P. Resorption of the mandibular condyle after injections of botulinum toxin A. Br J Oral Maxillofac Surg 2017;55(9):987–8.

49. Shinn JR, Nwabueze NN, Du L, et al. Treatment patterns and outcomes in botulinum therapy for patients with facial synkinesis. JAMA Facial Plast Surg 2019;21(3):244–51.

50. O'Rourke SP, Miller MQ. Predicting depressor anguli oris excision outcomes using local muscle block. Facial Plast Surg Aesthet Med 2022. https://doi. org/10.1089/fpsam.2022.0282.

51. Longino ES, Davis SJ, Landeen KC, et al. Chemodenervation of the posterior belly of the digastric muscle in facial synkinesis. Facial Plast Surg Aesthet Med 2022. https://doi.org/10.1089/fpsam.2022.0207.

52. Carruthers JDA, Glogau RG, Blitzer A. Facial aesthetics consensus group faculty. Advances in facial rejuvenation: botulinum toxin type A, hyaluronic acid dermal fillers, and combination therapies–consensus recommendations. Plast Reconstr Surg 2008;121(5 Suppl):5S–30S.

Volumizing Fillers for Skin
Selection Strategies

Victor G. Lacombe, MD

KEYWORDS

- Volumizing fillers • Hyaluronic acid • Biostimulatory fillers • Aesthetic • Injectable device
- Soft tissue augmentation

KEY POINTS

- Hydrophilicity is a key product factor to take into account when selecting a filler for a particular application.
- Hardness, or gel firmness, whether softer or firmer can create definition and lift or smooth out fine lines depending upon the desired effects.
- Cohesivity of a given hyaluronic product can aid in not only product lift capacity, but a natural appearance in high movement areas and is a gel property useful to understand in product selection.
- Biostimulation is an exciting property of fillers that can create longer lasting and global volumizing effects for patients able to grow their own collagen.

INTRODUCTION

From the moment of birth, the aging process weathers and beats on the skin resulting in collagen loss and thinning. Compounding on this is loss of volume, whether through fat loss, water loss, muscle or bone loss, and scarring. The overall effect is that the glow of youth is quick to fade and that thin-skinned humans are often quick to seek treatments to restore their appearance, symmetry or more youthful countenances. Modern cosmetic medicine has brought science to the table to aid in the pursuit of beauty and agelessness and volumizing fillers have become a part of that tool box.

HISTORY

To revolumize the aging face, injectable fillers have been a mainstay of clinical treatment for more than two decades in the United States and longer in Europe. For 20 years before that, bovine collagen was used as a dermal line filler, although its limitations included allergic reactions, skin testing, and short duration of action. The introduction of hyaluronic acid (HA), first as an animal extract and then as a human recombinant, transformed the practice of facial fillers. In 2003, Restylane was approved by the Food and Drug Administration (FDA) as a dermal filler for the nasolabial fold. Subsequently, a multitude of different HA, biostimulatory volumetric fillers, such as poly-L-lactic acid (PLLA), calcium hydroxyapatite, and a permanent filler, polymethyl methacrylate microspheres have been approved for a variety of indications.

DEFINITIONS

The largest category of volumizing filler is comprised of HA, which are cross-linked via a chemical cross-linker to stabilize the HA molecule. HA is a polysaccharide that is the main component of the ground substance or the extracellular matrix. The way that the HAs are differentiated is the concentration of HA, the degree of cross-linking, the resulting G′, the lift capacity, the cohesivity, or stretchability. These differentiators allow for a diverse array of clinical applications from skin boosting to reshaping bony structures.

PLLA, clinically approved as Sculptra and Sculptra Aesthetic in the United States,[1,2] essentially consists of small particles of a substance similar to an absorbable suture material

Artemedica, 1002 Mendocino Avenue, Sonoma County, Santa Rosa, CA 95401, USA
E-mail address: drlacombe@hotmail.com
Website: http://www.artemedica.com

Facial Plast Surg Clin N Am 31 (2023) 521–524
https://doi.org/10.1016/j.fsc.2023.05.009
1064-7406/23/© 2023 Elsevier Inc. All rights reserved.

suspended in a solution of water. These PLLA particles when injected under the skin stimulate a collagen-generating response that in turn thickens and firms the skin.

Calcium hydroxyapatite, also known as Radiesse, is a white paste-like filler that has components similar to native bone or teeth.[3] It can provide large-volume restorations and is best suited for thicker areas and not as well suited in areas with thin delicate structures, such as lip, tear trough, or where reversal may be needed.

Polymethyl methacrylate is the only permanent filler that is FDA approved at this time and the permanent component is mixed with resorbable HA to provide volume until native collagen is stimulated to form around the polymethyl methacrylate beads.[4] This product is FDA approved in the nasolabial fold.

DISCUSSION

The proper selection of soft tissue fillers is dependent on the location, depth of injection, and the degree of movement that the treatment area will be subjected to once the product is placed. Careful consideration of these factors plays a significant role in the success of achieving a natural and functional restoration or rejuvenation in a patient. Patient-specific factors are also important and include skin thickness and propensity for extracellular edema in the area of interest.[5]

Many types of corrections are categorized into deep/preperiosteal injections versus superficial/deep dermal or immediately subdermal injections meant to firm and thicken the actual dermis. One of the first areas of filler treatment was the nasolabial fold. This area was the target of many of the initial filler clinical trials because it afforded a built in control in the same subject and was easily reproducible and evaluated in person and by photography. The nasolabial fold is treated with a deep and a superficial technique of injection and thus is amenable to correction by multiple different types of filler with a variety of hydrological characteristics.

The best fillers for deep correction include those with greater G′ and/or lift capacities, which will sit on the periosteum and lift the skin and soft tissues. This author uses Juvederm Voluma XC, Volux, and Restylane Lyft primarily, but Restylane Defyne, Radiesse, and Sculptra are also used in this method. These are called the deeper fillers for reference purposes. Injection techniques could include deep depot or a peaking/cone-shaped injection as the needle is withdrawn from the bone.

If a more superficial technique is desired or indicated because of skin thickness or surface wrinkling, then a softer, thinner filler more likely to move with the expressions in this part of the face is better suited to the injections. Appropriate fillers include Juvederm Ultra or Ultra Plus, Restylane-L, Refyne, and RHA 2 or 3.

The treatment of fine lines and wrinkles and the use of fillers to create a skin boosting or hydrating effect for the skin requires an entirely different set of properties from the injectable agent in addition to different injection techniques. Generally lower concentration of HA in the filler and lower G′ are forgiving because they need to be placed very superficially in the mid-dermis to achieve the desired effects. Examples of these fillers are Redensity/RHA 1, SkinVive/Volite, Volbella, Vollure, RHA 2, and Restylane Silk. Techniques for achieving skin boosting are serial microboluses in the deep dermal plane in a gridlike pattern, cross hatching, or ferning. Care must be taken when filling an individual line not to place too much product in the superficial dermis as to avoid ridging and Tindal effects.

Treatment of the lip has become one of the most requested areas in the cosmetic arena in the last few years. Selection of the proper filler can aid in achieving a desirable outcome, although fashions do change with the time as to what style is considered desirable. Choosing a filler that will not be too hard and that can move naturally with expression is a logical goal. Maintaining and defining the vermillion border especially as the lip ages requires a filler with some degree of structural integrity and then providing soft fullness to the tubercles and body of the lip that has deflated with age or was never as full as desired is the next goal. The author's product of choice is Restylane Kysse. It provides a good balance for border definition, flexibility, and body fullness without stiffness. Juvederm Ultra XC does not provide as crisp a border. Restylane-L provides outstanding border definition, but is less plumping in the body of the lip. Often a firmer product is needed when addressing the melolabial folds or the downturned corners of the mouth because this skin and the muscles affecting the area are thicker and stronger than the lip structures.

Another area of the face that has gained popularity to rejuvenate with volumizing fillers is the cheeks. Two techniques lend themselves to proper filler results. The first technique is deep, depot injection on the bone or a midlevel injection in the subcutaneous level to round and smooth out wrinkles and reinflate. The deeper fillers, as mentioned previously, all mostly work for this purpose when injected along the zygoma and lateral midface. For the second technique, cannula injection or serial threading/fanning is performed in the subdermal plane or slightly deeper to fill the cheek.

The products suitable for this application include RHA 3 and 4, Voluma XC, Refyne, Contour, and Sculptra. Key injection pearls are to avoid infraorbital nerve and arteries as they exit the infraorbital foramen and to ensure that cheek filling for male clients is not too round or wide as to avoid feminizing the face unless that is a desired effect.

A related but more complicated anatomic area is the tear trough. More prone to edema and overfilling when treated, this arc along the infraorbital rim is frequently in need of volume restoration. The tear trough is rife with poorly executed attempts to correct the deformity, but is rewarding when properly corrected with filler. In this area, a lower degree of hydrophilicity is important, and the proper injection plane. Avoiding intramuscular injection, especially medially, avoids a lot of problems. The author has personally had to dissolve product injected in the medial third of the tear trough that was at the level of the orbicularis muscle 6 years after a single injection session because of excessive puffy edema. The only product specifically FDA approved for the tear trough is Juvederm Volbella XC. The injection plane for Volbella is clearly quite superficial and the product has low hydrophilicity. There have also been successful reports of Belotero in this area. The author's preferred injection technique is a periosteal depot injection at the top of the orbital rim with either Juvederm Voluma or Restylane Lyft-L. The use of a cannula is more comfortable for some injectors. This method using either of these products can slide under the orbital musculature and minimizes bruising after injection. The use of Hylacross Juvederm products and Radiesse and RHA is discouraged. The Hylacross products often induce chronic swelling, the Radiesse is too firm and cannot be dissolved in the case of improper placement or intravascular accident, and the RHA is meant for more superficial injection and being hydrophilic.

Between the eyes is a prominent facial subunit, the nose, which is often a surgical candidate, but can sometimes be temporarily disguised and reshaped with fillers. The nose frequently has convexities and concavities associated with its profile that lends itself to filling of those concavities to feign a more planar and often a smaller appearing overall projection. Artful placement of fill at the nasion and at the tip of the nose can change the entire shape of a nose. It can take a profile with a strong hump and a droopy tip and transform it into a nose that looks shorter, straight, and with a cute upturned tip within a matter of minutes. This assumes the proper patient selection, knowledge of anatomy, a skillful artist eye, and careful injection technique. The most common filler is the deep fillers for their properties the closest to

cartilage or bone yet higher safety profile. There is a risk of intravascular injection that could result in ischemic accidents, stroke, or blindness, therefore caution and expertise must be exercised when performing treatments in this area.

At the bottom of the face is another rewarding area for injection whether it is for weak anatomy, sagging jowls, or the loss of soft tissue support in the prejowl or angle of the mandible. Soft tissue augmentation with volumizing fillers can dramatically reshape the lower face. For the retrognathic patient, 2 to 3 mL of filler can create an immediate chin augmentation. Although not as permanent as a silastic implant the lack of downtime or need for surgery is tempting. Juvederm Voluma, Restylane Lyft, and Juvederm Volux have all been FDA indicated for use to augment the chin area. The high G′, high lift capacity fillers are the fillers of choice for this bone-simulating type of correction. Injection techniques include depot and superficial injection planes with the needle and cannula. Typically a combination technique centered primarily on the deep injection with a needle is preferred with shaping in the layer of the soft tissue above the mentalis muscle is the best. When hypognathia is truly the issue then blending the augmentation laterally onto the prejowl is usually important for a natural look.

Appreciation for a defined jawline has recently become more top of mind for patients, social media, cosmetic injectable companies, and providers. Jawline augmentation can take the form of restoring lost volume or creating a structure that never existed. Aging patients experience the draping of fat and skin over the mandible in the form of jowling and posterior mandibular and prejowl volume loss. Allergan validated a jawline definition scale to study and gain approval for Juvederm Volux for the improvement of the aging jawline. There exist others, often younger patients, who have weak mandibular projections at the angle and anteriorly who seek out sculpting with a volumizing filler for their jawlines. Before the approval of Juvederm Volux, the use of alternative deeper fillers was typical because the duplication of bony structure was the goal of augmentation. Depot bolus injection to the angle of the mandible creates lateral projection and sets the point from which the definition of the border of the mandible can be further augmented. From that point, lateral projection can be achieved at the angle and vertical definition up the ramus of the mandible. Using a cannula or a 27G needle sharper definition and molding of the body of the mandible can then occur anterior to the point of the angle to conceal any potential jowling. Caution is necessary anterior to the masseter muscle in the area of the antegonial notch and the facial artery. Deeper injection techniques are much riskier and aspiration essential, whereas a more superficial approach may be preferable. The full or ptotic jowl does not receive filler augmentation and the prejowl concavity is reached next as the correction moves anteriorly toward the mentum. Again, filling begins deep and along the inferior aspect of the mandible often with a cone-like technique to distribute product within the tissue. The ultimate goal is to create a smooth linear progression from the angle of the mandible forward to the front of the chin while defining a sharper definition of the jawline from the neck below when the injection is complete.

Although the jawline affords itself to a deep injection with a firm filler, an area like the décolletage, which is often sun damaged and wrinkled and thin, does not respond to a similar treatment. In fact most treatments even with thinner HA fillers have left the area lumpy, bumpy, and unsatisfactory. One treatment that has been useful is using dilute solutions of PLLA. A series of treatments can firm and thicken the skin and soften the wrinkles with movement, which are so bothersome to many women. A deep dermal or immediately subdermal injection plane is most desirable in this application. The consensus among key opinion leaders is that PLLA should be avoided in the neck area. Here skin boosters with ultra-thin HAs (SkinVive/Volite, RHA 1/Redensity) are used in a grid-like fashion to achieve wrinkle softening and texture improvement.

In an area with thicker skin, such as the buttocks, PLLA is effective at providing broad coverage at the superficial layer to firm and thicken where dimpling and divots occur because of cellulite.[6] The injection must be at a superficial level and not deep into the fat to see visible results for cellulite, but is satisfying for patient and provider. PLLA is also used in larger quantities in the gluteal region to achieve shaping and sculpting when volumizing is the goal. However, multiple sessions and 20 to 50 vials of product may be necessary to achieve real results. The advantages compared with surgical fat transfers include no need for a donor site, no risk of fat emboli, and utility in thinner patients without tangible donor locations. The level of the injection should be at the dermal subcutaneous junction. At this level thickening of the dermis is possible, which helps with the improvement of texture. Cellulite in the form of dimpling and deeper indents has been treated with moderate success with PLLA into the deep dermis and subdermal plane.

SUMMARY

There are a myriad of reasons that volume may need to be restored under the skin from trauma, birth defect, asymmetry, aging, weight loss, to medical conditions. There have evolved almost as many different methods and types of fillers as there are different types of needs that present themselves to clinicians treating the medical and cosmetic demands from patients. HA fillers offer a wide variety of options for skin volumization. Knowledge of the varying characteristics of the fillers is vital to the proper selection of the right filler and the right depth of application for that device. There are also instances when HAs are not the appropriate choice and where other fillers are better suited. Having an entire toolbox at a clinician's disposal is the practice for optimal outcomes.

CLINICS CARE POINTS

- Choose the right filler for the right application
- Deep fillers versus thinner superficial fillers
- Understand anatomy and filler properties

DISCLOSURE

The author has been a phase 3 clinical investigator for Galderma and Allergan/AbbVie. The author also served on advisory boards for Allergan/AbbVie, Alastin, and Galderma.

REFERENCES

1. Sculptra [prescribing information]. Bridgewater, NJ: Dermik Laboratories, a business of sanofi-aventis U.S. LLC; 2006.
2. Sculptra(r)Aesthetic [prescribing information]. Bridgewater, NJ: Dermik Laboratories; 2009.
3. Radiesse injectable implant [package insert]. Franksville, WI: BioForm Medical Inc; 2006.
4. Cohen S, Dover J, Monheit G, et al. Five-year safety and satisfaction study of PMMA-collagen in the correction of nasolabial folds. Dermatol Surg 2015; 41(Suppl 1):S302–13.
5. Kontis T, Lacombe V. Choosing the right filler. In: Cosmetic injection techniques. New York: Thieme; 2016. p. 101–6.
6. Swearingen A, Medrano K, Ferzli G, et al. Randomized Double-Blind Placebo-Controlled Study of Poly-L-Lactic acid for Treatment of Cellulite in the Lower Extremities. J Drugs Dermatol 2021;20(5):529–33.

Degradation Therapy with Collagenase and Deoxycholate

Louise McDonald, MB, BCh, BAO, BSc (Hons)[a],*, Lauren Hoffman, MD[b],
Anne Chapas, MD[b]

KEYWORDS

- Deoxycholate • Deoxycholic acid • ATX-101 • Kybella • Collagenase • Degradation therapy
- Submental fat • Non-invasive facial contouring

KEY POINTS

- Deoxycholate (deoxycholic acid) and collagenase are naturally occurring substances whose ability to degrade adipose tissue and collagen respectively has given rise to a variety of therapeutic applications.
- Degradation therapy in the form of deoxycholic acid offers a safe and efficacious non-invasive alternative to surgery for the reduction of submental fullness.
- The postulated mechanisms by which collagenase is of benefit in healing and reducing scar formation may result in new therapeutic applications in facial cosmetic treatments in the future.

INTRODUCTION

Deoxycholate (deoxycholic acid) and collagenase are naturally occurring substances whose ability to degrade adipose tissue and collagen respectively has given rise to a variety of therapeutic applications. This article will discuss the indications for the use of deoxycholic acid, primarily its well-established role in the non-surgical reduction of submental fat, with a focus on patient assessment, procedural technique, risks, pitfalls, and key clinical tips. It will also review the indications for collagenase therapy and its utility in the management of wound healing and scarring. Amidst the ever-increasing demand for minimally invasive cosmetic procedures,[1,2] it is important that physicians are appraised of the potential benefits, limitations, and risks of such degradation therapies when assessing patients who may elect for non-invasive therapeutic options for cosmetic concerns.

DEOXYCHOLIC ACID
Background

Deoxycholic Acid (DCA) is an endogenous secondary bile acid involved in the emulsification of dietary fat before subsequent absorption in the gastrointestinal system.[3] ATX-101 is the non-commercial name for the synthetic form of DCA and gained FDA approval in 2015 as an injectable drug for the treatment of moderate to severe submental convexity or fullness associated with submental fat (Kybella (USA), Belkyra (Europe, Canada, Australia, Kythera Biopharmaceuticals, Inc. (an affiliate of Allergan)).[4] ATX-101 offers a non-invasive alternative to manage unwanted pre-platysmal subcutaneous fat and improve mandibular definition.

Mechanism of Action

When injected into subcutaneous fat, ATX-101 causes adipocyte destruction by physically

[a] Department of Dermatology, Ulster Hospital, Upper Newtownards Road, Dundonald, Belfast, Northern Ireland BT16 1RH, UK; [b] Union Square Laser Dermatology, 19 Union Square West, 5th Floor, New York, NY 10003, USA
* Corresponding author.
E-mail address: louisemcdonald@doctors.org.uk

Facial Plast Surg Clin N Am 31 (2023) 525–533
https://doi.org/10.1016/j.fsc.2023.05.005
1064-7406/23/© 2023 Elsevier Inc. All rights reserved.

disrupting the cell membrane and causing necrosis, inflammation, and subsequent fat clearance.[5-8] Lipid liberation during this process results in raised plasma lipid levels akin to a post-prandial and non-clinically relevant level.[8,9] When injected subcutaneously, ATX-101 is excreted in the enterohepatic circulation together with the endogenous bile pool.[6] ATX-101 is relatively selective for adipose tissue with the preferential destruction of adipocytes and this is postulated to be due to a relative absence of binding proteins in adipose tissue which would otherwise neutralize and inactivate ATX-101 in other tissues.[5,7] Following adipocytolysis, a mild inflammatory response ensues with remission and fibroblast proliferation evident and observed histologically by day 28.[10]

Summary of Clinical Trial Evidence

Prior to FDA approval, ATX-101 was extensively evaluated over many years in multiple Phase I to III clinical trials and its safety and efficacy was validated in no less than 4 randomized, double-blind, placebo-controlled Phase III clinical trials. These included 2 identical large-scale European studies conducted across 37 centers in Europe and the UK and 2 conducted across 35 centers in North America (REFINE 1 and REFINE 2)).[3,10-13] The trials enrolled adult patients aged 18-65 with moderate to severe submental fat who were randomized to receive 1 or 2 mg/cm2 of ATX-101 in up to 4 treatment sessions with 28-day treatment intervals.

Objective analysis of the severity of submental convexity and efficacy of ATX-101 was performed using a validated 5-point Clinician-Reported Submental Fat Rating Scale (CR-SMFRS),[13] caliper assessment and a patient-reported Subject Self-Rating Scale (SSRS)). Subjects were required to demonstrate stable body weight for at least 6 months prior to inclusion and have a BMI less than 30 kg/m^2 in the European and less than 40 kg/m^2 in the US and Canadian studies. Exclusion criteria were previous treatment for submental fat, recent aesthetic treatment of chin or neck, skin laxity or trauma in the area, prominent platysmal bands, and patients with any other cause of enlargement in the submental area or co-morbid medical conditions that may affect full participation in analyses or consent.

Follow-up evaluation for all RCTs took place 12 weeks after the final treatment. All trials confirmed the efficacy of 2 mg/cm^2 ATX-101 dosing by meeting the co-primary endpoints of an improvement of one or more points from baseline using the CR-SMFRS and a final patient-reported satisfaction score of 4 (slightly satisfied) to 6 (extremely satisfied) on the SSRS. Data suggest that clinically meaningful results are achieved within 2-4 treatment sessions. The REFINE trial data also demonstrated a greater reduction in submental volume in 225 patients treated with ATX-101 versus placebo in objective MRI analyses.[11] Rigorous safety data reported in the trials confirmed that the majority of adverse events were of mild-moderate intensity, short-lived, and resolved within the treatment interval time-frame. The most common were related to the injection area and included injection-site pain, bruising, swelling, numbness, and induration and erythema. REFINE data also reported an incidence of marginal mandibular nerve paresis of 4.3% in patients given ATX-101 versus 0.4% of those receiving placebo and confirmed that such paresis was mild and temporary[11] but the authors highlighted the importance of physician training and knowledge of the relevant anatomy in mitigating against adverse events.

Submental Fat Contouring using Deoxycholic Acid

Patient selection

The well-documented positive effect of ATX-101 on submental fullness represents a welcome additional non-invasive option in the quest for an aesthetically pleasing neck. Features of such a neckline include a well-defined mandibular border, a cervicomental angle of 105°-120° with visible anatomical landmarks of sternocleidomastoid, thyroid cartilage, and sub-hyoid depression. Many variables contribute to a perceived suboptimal neckline. Individual patient anatomical features such as chin and hyoid bone location can impact cervicomental angle and factors such as submandibular gland and soft tissue ptosis, mandibular atrophy, skin laxity, and subcutaneous adipose tissue can all obscure the mandibular line.[14,15] It has been reported that the ideal cervicomental angle in 126° and 121° in adult males and females respectively.[16] A square shaped jaw has been conventionally associated with attractiveness for males[17,18] and Shridharani and Behr published valuable insights from their practice confirming that contour loss of the jawline as a result of submental fullness is a major aesthetic concern for men. Pre-treatment clinical evaluation and appropriate patient selection, however, are crucial to optimize efficacy as well as reduce the risk of adverse outcomes.

A pragmatic and insightful best practice article by Teller and colleagues[10] helpfully detailed the recommendations of a convention of USA physicians experienced in the use of ATX-101 in submental contouring.[10] A standardized physical assessment is recommended prior to any ATX-101 treatment to delineate anatomical landmarks and screen for problems. First, one should document the location of any submental fat. Patients with moderate or greater submental fullness should be deemed appropriate candidates when fullness is due to preplatysmal or subplatysmal fat. This can be assessed by having the patient flex the platysmal muscle while palpating the preplatysmal fat pad in the submental region. Preplatysmal fat can be grasped and palpated above the platysma with simultaneous platysmal engagement.[14]

Patients should also be evaluated for other causes of submental fullness including thyromegaly, cervical or submandibular lymphadenopathy, salivary gland enlargement, a low or anterior hyoid bone, or digastric muscle strength.[10] Patients should also carefully assess swallowing to rule out dysphagia, as well as, smile symmetry to assess marginal mandibular nerve function.[14]

The expert panel reminded practitioners that patients with severe laxity or excess sub-platysmal fat may be more suited to alternative management strategies or a combination approach. For example, those with long or wide platysmal bands will have suboptimal outcomes with ATX-101 therapy and may require follow-up treatment with neuromodulation and/or surgical intervention.[10] Contraindications to ATX-101 injection include injection-site infection, pregnancy, aged under 18.[5] Patients with previous submental or anterior cervical surgery, facial nerve paralysis or dysphagia are not ideal candidates for ATX-101 treatment in this area.[14] Treatments should be spaced at least 4 weeks apart with an interval of 6-8 weeks being reported as optimal by experienced clinicians[10,14] (**Fig. 1**).

It is important to counsel patients about the likely outcomes and time course for improvement prior to administering ATX-101 to ensure expectations are managed appropriately.[10,19] Baseline and post-procedure photography is also recommended to objectively monitor progress.[10] **Fig. 1** demonstrates baseline and follow-up imaging for a real-world patient receiving ATX-101 therapy for submental fullness.

Procedure for Administration of ATX-101 for the Treatment of Submental Fullness

Technique
Once mutually agreed treatment goals are decided, the target treatment area should be prepped.[14]

1. The patient should be positioned comfortably in a semi-upright position, with the head reclined slightly and resting on a headrest.
2. Clean skin thoroughly with antiseptic solution and with surgical pen. Mark anatomic boundaries of preplatysmal fat as follows:
   a. Mark inferior mandibular border along the length of jawline.
   b. Below the mandibular border, mark a line 1.0 to 1.5 cm. This outlines a zone to avoid treatment where the marginal mandibular nerve may course.
   c. Mark the hyoid bone inferiorly.
   d. Draw a line vertically as a continuation from labio-mandibular fold, which creates lateral boundaries of preplatysmal fat.

Injections should be spaced 1 cm apart by using the included temporary tattoo grid, superimposed onto the treatment area (**Fig. 2**). The volume (in milliliters) of DCA needed can be calculated by counting the number of tattoo grid injection points within the boundaries divided by 5 (as 0.2 mL is delivered with each injection).

A dosage of 2 mg/cm^2 of ATX-101 should be injected perpendicularly into the "pinchable" preplatysmal subcutaneous fat in the submental area with a 30 gauge 0.5-inch needle. Up to 50 injections of 0.2 mL each to a depth of 0.25 to 0.5 inches and spaced 1 cm apart on the grid (up to a total volume of 10 mL) may be administered.[5] Avoid injecting too superficially, which can lead to necrosis. The CONTOUR trial data evaluating real-world administration reported a relatively stable mean volume administration of 3.2 to 3.5 mL/treatment.[20]

Important risks and adverse events As with any clinical intervention, comprehensive counselling is vital to ensure patients are fully informed before deciding to proceed with treatment. Although ATX-101 is usually very well tolerated, a variety of side effects have been reported both in trial data and real-world practice.

Common treatment-related side effects
The most common side effects include pain, swelling, bruising, numbness, erythema, induration, nausea, paresthesia, pruritus, and subcutaneous nodule formation.[10–13] These were usually localized to the injection site, transient and resolved without intervention. Pain reduction measures have been well-documented by previous reviews and include the application of cold compresses, ice, topical and injectable local anesthetic agents, oral analgesia such as acetaminophen pre-procedure, antihistamines, and mechanical support in the form of post-treatment chin strapping.[19,21] Although caution with the

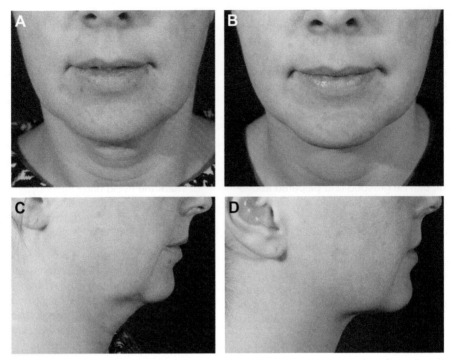

Fig. 1. Treatment efficacy of submental fullness with deoxycholic acid. (*A&C*). Baseline frontal and side views, respectively. (*B&D*), response after one treatment at 4-months follow-up of frontal and side views, respectively.

combination injection of deoxycholic acid with lidocaine or steroid has been advocated due to potential safety and efficacy concerns and theoretical impeding of collagen formation,[18] in the authors' experience injection of buffered lidocaine has not impacted clinical outcomes and has resulted in a more comfortable and positive patient experience. After gridding, 0.1 mL of buffered 1% lidocaine is injected into each treatment point prior to DCA injection.

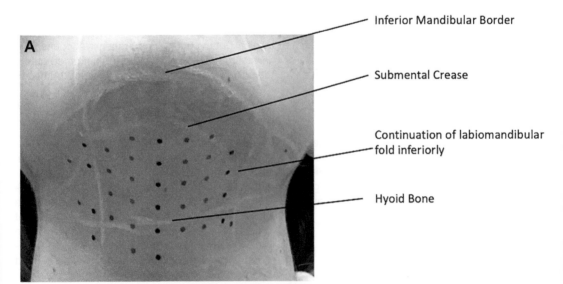

Fig. 2. Marked anatomic boundaries of preplatysmal fat with temporary tattoo grid markings prior to injection with Deoxycholic Acid. Borders include the submental crease superiorly, caudal continuation of labiomandibular folds laterally, and hyoid bone inferiorly. Avoid treating in the gap between inferior mandibular border and submental crease, as the risk to injuring the Marginal Mandibular Nerve is greater in this region.

Less common adverse effects

Metzger and colleagues,[22] conducted a review of uncommon adverse effects of deoxycholic acid injection, including dysphagia, alopecia, and skin necrosis. Factors that increase the risk of such adverse events were identified as well as the importance of recognizing these events in our own patients and those treated elsewhere.

Dysphagia has been reported as an adverse effect of ATX-101 injection with an incidence of 1.9% in the clinical trial data and much less frequently in real-world data (0.2%).[11,23] Such swallowing difficulty is felt to result from localized swelling in the injection area and all cases resolved spontaneously.

Alopecia following ATX-101 injection was reported in the REFINE trials as a less common and transient occurrence (0.4%). There have been a small number of case reports documenting localized and non-scarring alopecia within the treated area which resolved over time.[24–26] One case report, however, documented alopecia after submental area injection which was diffuse initially but then became persistent and patchy with minimal regrowth.[27] The mechanism for developing alopecia post–ATX-101 injection is unclear but histopathological analysis in one case suggested a telogen effluvium phenomenon.[26]

Skin necrosis resulting from inadvertent vascular injury following deoxycholic acid injection is rare, with four case reports in the literature.[28–31] Injection site pain and purpura development were immediate with pain presenting as key features. Scarring was a notable adverse outcome as a result of the cutaneous inflammation induced by vascular injury. Injecting too superficially increases the risk of such skin necrosis.[10]

Marginal mandibular nerve damage

Careful delineation of anatomical landmarks in the cervico-mental area is vital to ensure the safe administration of ATX-101 and, in particular, avoid the risk of injury to the marginal mandibular nerve (MMN).[6,14,32] This nerve courses under the mandible before running superiorly to innervate lower facial muscles including the lip depressors. Damage of the MMN can result in temporary asymmetry of smile and paresis (**Fig. 3**). REFINE data reported a 4.3% risk of MMN damage in patients treated with ATX-101[11] and the CONTOUR trial reported a lower risk 0.2%[22] suggesting this occurs less frequently in real-world practice. Shridharani also published data from a 2-year follow-up assessment of 100 patients undergoing deoxycholic acid injection for neck contouring and only 2 experienced MMN paresis.[33] The exit point at which the MMN traverses the mandible

can be palpated at the antegonial notch at the anterior border of the clenched masseter. Avoiding injection into a 1.0 to 1.5 cm zone marked between the inferior mandibular border and submental crease reduces the risk of inadvertently injecting in the submandibular course of the MMN.[14,34] The target pre-platysmal adipose tissue should be clearly marked including the inferior border of the mandible, hyoid bone and inferior extension of the line of the labio-mandibular folds to define lateral borders.

Best clinical practice guidance also reminds physicians undertaking ATX-101 injection treatment to be mindful of pseudo-MMN symptoms as a result of injury to platysma causing muscle demyelination and inflammation. To avoid this, physicians should ensure that injections are not administered too deep.[10,35]

Non-submental Indications for Deoxycholate Therapy

As discussed, DCA in the form of ATX-101[6] (Kybella), is currently only FDA-approved as an injectable for the minimally invasive treatment of submental fat reduction with robust evidence documenting its efficacy for this indication. Other applications harnessing the contouring effects of deoxycholic acid in other regions of the body are used "off-label" but have been reported with similar safety and patient satisfaction outcomes. A number of potential alternative injection sites were outlined in a recent review article[36] and include the jowl, face and chin, bra line adiposity, gluteo-trochanteric region, painful piezogenic pedal papules, paradoxical adipose hyperplasia following cryolipolysis, HIV/HAART-associated lipodystrophy of the buccal fat pad, lipoma and xanthelasma although patient numbers were small.[36] The reviewers also suggested the intradermal injection of ATX-101 for periorbital xanthelasma was reported in 2 patients[37] without complications and further studies were encouraged. It would be important to be aware of potential complications of post-treatment swelling following injection in the periocular region. Shridharani published cadaver dissection study results delineating clear surface markings to guide the safe injection of ATX-101 for excess jowl fat on an "off-label" basis.[38] He discusses the importance of identifying an individual's jowling mechanism to ensure they are an appropriate candidate for ATX-101 and states that visible focal fullness and palpable subcutaneous fat should be present at the jowl in the suitable candidate. He also comments how better skin integrity in the younger patient may confer less risk of skin laxity following isolated subcutaneous fat reduction and that

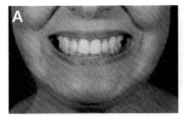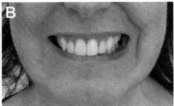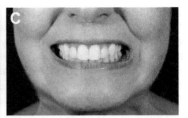

Fig. 3. Marginal Mandibular Nerve Injury following treatment with Kybella. Injury to the marginal mandibular nerve on the right side, (*A*) One day after treatment, (*B*) 1 month after treatment, (*C*) 2 months after treatment.

some patients may be better suited to surgical rejuvenation.

An interesting article by Sykes and colleagues[39] suggests additional non-FDA approved applications for ATX-101 such as anterior and posterior axillary fat, upper arm, medial and lateral knee fat, and subcutaneous abdominal fat. The authors highlight, however, the limiting factors of ATX-101 such as the cost and volume required to treat larger body areas which would need to be considered when counselling patients.[39]

COLLAGENASE
Background

Collagenase, first identified in 1962, has been used in various laboratory and therapeutic settings over the years. It is an enzyme that breaks down peptide bonds in types I, II, III, and IV collagen without disrupting the cell membrane. Collagenase enzymes come from both microbial cells and animal tissues. Pathogenic microorganisms, mainly *Clostridium histiolyticum (C.histiolyticum),* have been approved by the FDA for breakdown of the cord-like contractures in Dupuytren's disease, as well as, treatment for Peyronie's disease. It has also been used in the promotion of wound healing and debridement, particularly in the management of burns.[40]

Collagenase clostridium histolyticum-aaes (CCH-aaes) in the injectable product QWO™ (Endo International PLC) was granted FDA approval for the treatment of moderate to severe cellulite in the buttocks of adult women in 2020. Injection of CCH-aaes in areas of cellulite related contour changes causes enzymatic release of pathogenic collagen-rich septae to improve cellulite-associated depressions and skin texture.[41] CCH-aaes was also found to stimulate neocollagenesis and reorganize subcutaneous adipose tissue into smaller and more homogenous fat lobules.[41] Injectable CCH-aaes was subsequently withdrawn from the market following concerns about treatment-related bruising and longer-term skin discoloration.[42] Their open-label study APHRODITE, designed to evaluate injection-related bruising, is scheduled for completion this year.[43]

Mechanism of Action in Wound and Scar Management

Collagenase enzymes can be a useful treatment option for wound healing and burns. When used in wound healing, collagenase can remove the necrotic tissue in the wound area, while sparing healthy tissue.[40] In vivo wound healing studies on swine[44] have demonstrated that Clostridial collagenase in growth media induced keratinocyte response to injury, along with, epithelial cell proliferation and migration to promote wound healing. Collagenase is already approved by the FDA for the treatment of burns and has been found to heal burn wounds faster than the standard treatment.[40] When compared to the surgical management of burn wounds, treatment with *C. histolytica* shortened hospital stay time and the need for subsequent surgery and transfusion in partial layer burns.[45]

Studies have also examined the potential role of collagenase in the management of keloid and hypertrophic scarring. In a pilot study, Kang and colleagues[46] found that the intra-lesional injection of pure collagenase into keloid and hypertrophic scars produced only a transient decrease in keloid scar volume. The treatment was ultimately deemed ineffective in reducing scar volume as both keloidal and hypertrophic scars returned back to baseline at 6-month follow-up. Limitations of this study included a small sample size of 7 patients, and only 5 of these 7 received more than one injection. Furthermore, none of the patients completed the final follow-up at 2 years. Other studies are necessary to further evaluate this application. A pilot study in 2011 evaluated the effects of a collagenase ointment in a rabbit ear animal model for the prevention of hypertrophic scars. The authors found that collagenase-treated wounds developed scars with less hypertrophy than untreated scars as measured by the total area of scar and scar elevation index.[47]

There is a paucity of data regarding the use of collagenase degradation therapy in facial cosmetic treatments but the postulated mechanisms by which it may help promote wound healing and reduce scar formation may result in new therapeutic applications in the future. At the time of publication, no clinical indication for facial treatment with collagenase has FDA approval. Larger and more robust studies are required with clinical data to further explore its efficacy and potential facial aesthetic applications.

SUMMARY

Degradation therapy in the form of deoxycholic acid is both a safe and efficacious non-invasive option in the armamentarium of the facial aesthetic practitioner. The robust evidence-base and wealth of documented real-world clinical experience have deemed ATX-101 a first-in-class injectable drug for the reduction of submental fat as an alternative to liposuction or surgery. With the destruction of unwanted adipose tissue by ATX-101, a subsequent wound healing response ensues to create a more durable improvement in the submental profile. The offer of sustained, reproducible, long-term results, with non-recurrence of the degraded substance combined with the ease and convenience of an office-based treatment with limited recovery time will continue to make degradation therapies a popular choice for both patients and providers.

CLINICS CARE POINTS

- Appropriate patient selection prior to the use of deoxycholic acid in submental fat reduction is crucial to ensure the best clinical outcomes
- A detailed knowledge of facial structures and key anatomical landmarks is vital to minimize the risk of injection-related adverse events such as marginal mandibular nerve injury.
- Careful delineation of the treatment area and marking of injection points helps ensure an adequate and appropriately spaced deoxycholic acid volume is administered
- As with all aesthetic treatments, managing patient expectations and agreeing individual treatment goals at the outset is of utmost importance.

DISCLOSURE

Dr L. McDonald has no conflicts of interest to declare. Dr L. Hoffman has no conflicts of interest to declare. Dr A. Chapas is a speaker and investigator for AbbVie, and has received honorarium for participating in advisory boards. She was also previously an investigator for Endo Pharmaceuticals.

REFERENCES

1. American Society of Dermatologic Surgery. 2021 ASDS Consumer survey on cosmetic dermatology procedures. Available at: https://www.asds.net/medical-professionals/practice-resources/consumer-survey-on-cosmetic-dermatologic-procedures. Accessed November 7th 2022.
2. American Society of Plastic Surgeons: Plastic Surgery Statistics Report 2020. Available at: https://www.plasticsurgery.org/documents/News/Statistics/2020/plastic-surgery-statistics-full-report-2020.pdf. Accessed November 7th 2022.
3. Ascher B, Hoffman K, Walker P, et al. Efficacy, patient-reported outcomes and safety profile of ATX-101 (deoxycholic acid), an injectable drug for the reduction of unwanted submental fat: results from a phase III, randomized, placebo-controlled study. J Eur Acad Dermatol Venereol 2014;28:1707–15.
4. Dayan SH, Humphrey A, Jones MD, et al. Overview of ATX-101 (Deoxycholic Acid Injection): a nonsurgical approach for reduction of submental fat. Dermatol Surg 2016;42(Suppl 1):S263–70.
5. Thuangtong R, Bentow JJ, Knopp K, et al. Tissue-selective effects of injected deoxycholate. Dermatol Surg 2010;36:899–908.
6. Kybella [package insert]. Irvine, Calif: Allergan USA, Inc.; 2020.
7. Rotunda AM. Injectable treatments for adipose tissue: terminology, mechanism and tissue interaction. Lasers Surg Med 2009;41:714–20.
8. Walker P, Lee D. Open-label pharmacokinetic study to evaluate lipid levels in the blood following injections of ATX-101 (synthetically derived sodium deoxycholate). JAAD 2013;68(4):AB1.
9. Ascher B, Fellman J, Monheit G. ATX-101 (deoxycholic acid injection) for reduction of submental fat. Expet Rev Clin Pharmacol 2016;9:1131–43.
10. Teller CF, Chin A, Chesnut AD, et al. Best Clinical Practices with ATX-101 for submental fat reduction: patient-related factors and physician considerations. Plast Reconstructr Surg Glob Open 2021;9:e3668.
11. Humphrey S, Sykes J, Kantor J, et al. ATX-101 for reduction of submental fat: a phase III randomized controlled trial. Dermatol Surg 2016;75:788–97.
12. Rzany B, Griffiths T, Lippert S, et al. Reduction of unwanted submental fat with ATX-101 (deoxycholic acid), an adipocytolytic injectable treatment: results from a phase III, randomized, placebo-controlled study. Br J Dermatol 2014;170:445–53.
13. McDiarmid J, Ruiz JB, Lee D, et al. Results from a pooled analysis of two european, randomized,

placebo-controlled, phase 3 studies of ATX-101 for the pharmacologic reduction of excess submental fat. Aesthetic Plast Surg 2014;38:849–60.

14. Hurst EA, Dietert JB. Nonsurgical treatment of submental fullness. Advances in Cosmetic Surgery 2018;1:1–15.

15. Fedok FG, Lighthall JG. Evaluation and treatment planning for the aging face patient. Facial Plast Surg Clin North Am 2022;30:277–90.

16. Sommerville JM, Sperry TP, BeGole EA. Morphology of the submental and neck region. Int J Adult Orthodon Orthognath Surg 1988;3:97–106.

17. Goodman GJ, Subramanian M, Sutch S, et al. Beauty from the neck up: introduction to the special issue. Dermatol Surg 2016;42(Suppl 1):S260–2.

18. Shridharani S, Behr K. ATX-101 (doexycholic acid injection) treatment in men: insights from our clinical experience. Dermatol Surg 2017;43:S225–30.

19. Fagien A, McChesney P, Subramanian S, et al. Prevention and management of injection-related adverse effects in facial aesthetics: considerations for ATX-101 (deoxycholic acid injection) treatment. Dermatol Surg 2016;42:S300–4.

20. Behr K, Kavah CM, Munavalli G, et al. ATX-101 (deoxycholic acid injection) leads to clinically meaningful improvement in submental fat: final data from CONTOUR. Dermatol Surg 2020;16:639–45.

21. Dover JS, Kenkel JM, Carruthers A, et al. Management of patient experience with ATX-101 (deoxycholic acid injection) for reduction of submental fat. Dermatol Surg 2016;42:S288–99.

22. Metzger KC, Crowley EL, Kadlubowska D, et al. Uncommon adverse effects of deoxycholic acid injection for submental fullness: beyond the clinical trials. J Cutan Med Surg 2020;24(6):619–24.

23. Palm MD, Schlessinger J, Callender VD, et al. Final data from the condition of submental fullness and treatment outcomes registry (CONTOUR). J Drugs Dermatol JDD 2019;18:10–8.

24. Grady B, Porphirio F, Rokhsar C. Submental alopecia at deoxycholic acid injection site. Dermatol Surg 2017;43(8):1105–8.

25. Wambier CG. Alopeica em barba causada por desoxicolato para tratamiento de gordura submentoniana. Surg Cosmet Dermatol 2017;9(3):259–60.

26. Sebaratnam DF, Wong XL, Kim L, et al. Alopecia following deoxycholic acid treatment for submental adiposity. JAMA Facial Plast Surg 2019;21(6):571–2.

27. Souyoul S, Gioe O, Emerson A, et al. Alopecia after injection of ATX-101 for reduction of submental fat. JAAD Case Reports 2017;3:250–2.

28. Riswold K, Flynn V. A cautionary tale: a vascular event with deoxycholic acid injection. Dermatol Surg 2018;44(6):887–9.

29. McKay C, Price C, Pruett L. Vascular injury after deoxycholic acid injection. Dermatol Surg 2019;45(2):306–9.

30. Sachdev D, Mohammadi T, Fabi SG. Deoxycholic acid-induced skin necrosis: prevention and management. Dermatol Surg 2018;44(7):1037–9.

31. Ramirez MR, Marinaro RE, Warthan ML, et al. Permanent cutaneous adverse events after injection with deoxycholic acid. Dermatol Surg 2019;45(11):1432–4.

32. Kenkel JM, Jones DH, Fagien S. Anatomy of the cervicomental region: insights from an anatomy laboratory ad roundtable discussion. Dermatol Surg 2016;42:S282–7.

33. Shridharani SM. Real-world experience with 100 consecutive patients undergoing neck contouring with ATX-101 (deoxycholic acid): an updated report with a 2-year analysis. Dermatol Surg 2019;45:1285–93.

34. Deeks ED. Deoxycholic acid: a review in submental fat contouring. Am J Clin Dermatol 2016;17:701–7.

35. Sorenson E, Chesnut C. Marginal mandibular versus pseudo-marginal mandibular nerve injury with submandibular deoxycholic acid injection. Dermatol Surg 2018;44(5):733–5.

36. Sung CT, Lee A, Choi F, et al. Non-submental applications of injectable deoxycholic acid: a systematic review. J Drugs Dermatol 2019;18(7):675–80.

37. Patel J, Ranjit-Reeves R, Woodward J. Recurrent xanthelasmas treated with intralesional deoxycholic acid. Dermatol Surg 2020;46(6):847–8.

38. Shridharani SM. Novel surface anatomic landmarks of the jowl to guide treatment with ATX-101. Plast Reconstr Surg Glob Open 2019;7:e2459.

39. Sykes JM, Allak A, Klink B. Future applications of deoxycholic acid in body contouring. J Drugs Dermatol 2017;16(1):43–6.

40. Alipour H, Raz A, Zakeri A, et al. Therapeutic applications of collagenase (metalloproteases): a review. Asian Pac J Trop Biomed 2016;6(11):975–81.

41. Bass LS, Kaufman-Janette J, Joseph JH, et al. Collagenase Clostridium Histolyticum-aaes for Treatment of Cellulite: A Pooled Analysis of Two Phase-3 Trials. Plast Reconstr Surg Glob Open 2022;10(5):e4306.

42. Endo International plc. Press Release. Available at: https://investor.endo.com/news-releases/news-release-details/endo-cease-production-and-sale-qwor-collagenase-clostridium. Accessed December 24, 2022.

43. Study of Different Interventions to Reduce Bruising Following CCH-Ases Treatment for Cellulite of the Buttocks (APHRODITE). Available at: https://clinicaltrials.gov/ct2/show/NCT05419505. Accessed January 26, 2023.

44. Riley KN, Herman I. Collagenase promotes the cellular responses to injury and wound healing in vivo. J Burns Wounds 2005;4:112–24.

45. McCallon SK, Weir D, Lantis JC 2nd. Optimizing wound bed preparation with collagenase enzymatic debridement. J Am Coll Clin Wound Spec 2015;6(1–2):14–23.

46. Kang N, Sivakumar B, Sanders R. Intra-lesional injections of collagenase are ineffective in the treatment of keloid and hypertrophic scars. J Plast Reconstr Aesthet Surg 2006;59(7):693–9.

47. Jia S, Zhao Y, Law M. The effects of collagenase ointment on the prevention of hypertrophic scarring in a rabbit ear scarring model: a pilot study. Wounds 2011;23(6):160–5.

Antiaging Effects of Topical Defensins

Arman Danielian, MD, MS[a], Marie Danielian, PharmD[b], Melodyanne Y. Cheng, MS[c], Jason Burton, MA[d], Peter S. Han, MD[a], Rhorie P.R. Kerr, MD, FACS[a],*

KEYWORDS

- Defensins • LGR6+ stem cells • Skin aging • Aesthetics • Dermatology • Rhytids

KEY POINTS

- Defensins stimulate LGR6+ stem cells, which sit just above the hair follicle bulge in the basal epidermal layer of the skin.
- Studies have demonstrated improvements in skin elasticity, skin moisture content, transepidermal water loss, pigmentation, pores, and wrinkles of the face and body after exposure to topical defensins.
- Research on the antiaging effects of topical defensins is in the early stages, and larger studies will be needed to generalize the results.

INTRODUCTION

A wide variety of antiaging products exist, all focusing on the common goal of alleviating the first and most outwardly visible signs of the aging process, specifically changes to skin morphology and physiology.[1,2] Current antiaging skincare products include a variety of organic and inorganic compounds, ranging from the extremely popular hyaluronic acid and other antioxidants (vitamins, polyphenols, and flavonoids) to cell regulators (retinols, peptides, hormones, and botanicals), and even injected nanoparticles.[3–5] However, both plant-based nonspecific growth factors and cell regulators, such as retinols, have raised concerns about side effects, particularly at higher exposure doses, highlighting the need for more targeted alternatives to combat dermal aging.[6,7]

Quintessentially discovered in 1961 by Till and McCulloch, multipotent stem cells have since demonstrated key applications in regenerative medicine.[8] Stem cell therapy plays an integral role in the treatment of a variety of pathologies, including hematological malignancies while also demonstrating experimental promise in many other areas, including heart failure, human immunodeficiency virus (HIV), and spinal cord injury.[9–12] In the context of aging and age-related dysfunctions, yet another important up-and-coming application of stem cell therapy is the use of stem cells to combat dermal aging.[13]

As biological aging is an intricate process influenced by both extrinsic and intrinsic factors, leveraging the pathophysiology behind dermal signaling pathways can help develop optimized treatments that target skin rejuvenation while hopefully minimizing the associated side effects and concerns associated with some of the more common antiaging products on the market. Photodamaged and other extrinsic or intrinsic aging factors may result in telomere-based deoxyribonucleic acid (DNA) responses, cellular senescence, inflammatory infiltrates, decreased/fragmented collagen, and increased matrix-degrading metalloproteases.[14,15] On histopathology, these aging changes manifest as thinning of the epidermis, flattening of the dermal–epidermal junction, an increasing type III collagen-to-type I

[a] Department of Head and Neck Surgery, David Geffen School of Medicine at UCLA, 200 Medical Plaza, Suite 550, Los Angeles, CA 90095, USA; [b] Independent Researcher, 200 Medical Plaza, Suite 550, Los Angeles, CA 90095, USA; [c] David Geffen School of Medicine at UCLA, 10833 Le Conte Ave, Los Angeles, CA 90095, USA; [d] University of California Los Angeles, 200 Medical Plaza, Suite 550, Los Angeles, CA 90095, USA
* Corresponding author. 200 Medical Plaza Driveway Suite 550, Los Angeles, CA 90095.
E-mail address: rkerr@mednet.ucla.edu

Facial Plast Surg Clin N Am 31 (2023) 535–546
https://doi.org/10.1016/j.fsc.2023.05.010
1064-7406/23/© 2023 Elsevier Inc. All rights reserved.

collagen ratio, lessening of basal cell proliferative ability, and hyperplasia of the sebaceous glands.[16–19] Phenotypically, these changes correlate with skin dryness, sallowness, wrinkle formation and depth, loss of elasticity, and telangiectasia and purpura formation.[19]

Recently, topical applications of antimicrobial peptides (AMPs) called defensins have shown promise in various clinical studies targeting the signs of dermal aging. Unlike retinols and other antiaging products, defensins, which are cationic peptides characterized by six cysteine residues and stabilized by three disulfide bridges, target a specific subtype of stem cells that do not divide throughout life.[20] This subtype, known as Leucine Rich Repeat Containing G Protein-Coupled Receptor 6 (LGR6+) stem cells, sits just above the hair follicle bulge in the basal epidermal layer of the skin and creates the entire epidermis and appendages early in utero; then, they remain dormant until they are activated by the healing cascade unleashed by a skin wound.[21–23] Defensins first demonstrated promise in augmenting wound healing in mice.[24] Although the ability of these defensin peptides to activate the epidermal basal stem cell layer and induce production of new basal stem cells and keratinocytes in wound healing has been well studied on a biological level, the application of alpha and beta defensin peptides has recently shown promising results for improving markers of aging skin as antiaging topicals.[13,25] Here, the authors conduct a thorough review of the literature and focus on the role of topical applications of defensins in combating dermal aging.

METHODS
Search Strategy

This systematic review was performed with adherence to The Preferred Reporting Items for Systematic Review and Meta-Analysis (PRISMA) guidelines. A literature search was conducted by a medical librarian (JB) on National Institutes of Health (NIH), Embase, Cochrane, and Web of Science. The search strategy with medical subject headings (MeSH) terms used in the NIH database is displayed in **Box 1**. This search strategy was replicated in the remaining medical databases with equivalent keywords and phrases.

Study Selection

The de-duplicated studies were screened by two independent reviewers (AD and MD). Articles were identified as relevant and eligible for full-text article analysis based on population,

inclusion, comparison, outcome inclusion criteria discussed below:

Patients: Adults (over the age of 18 years) free of preexisting dermatologic or systemic disorders (ie, systemic lupus erythematosus, rheumatoid arthritis, HIV, atopic dermatitis/eczema); *Intervention*: application of topical alpha-defensin or beta-defensin-containing compound to skin including face or body; *Comparison*: pretreatment and posttreatment skin characteristics; *Outcome*: subjective and objective changes in skin composition including skin thickness, skin roughness, hydration, transepidermal water loss (TEWL), pores, wrinkles, and skin tone; *Study design*: all randomized controlled trials (RCTs) and prospective studies were included in the study.

Exclusion criteria: Articles not available in English, lack of full-text availability and articles not assessing the effects of topical defensins on skin composition.

This review did not require Institutional Review Board approval as it did not constitute human subject research.

RESULTS

A total of 277 studies were identified following the search strategy. After de-duplication, 137 studies remained. Following title/abstract screening then full-text review, three studies were deemed eligible for inclusion in this study. A flow diagram depicting study selection process is displayed in **Fig. 1**.

Summary of Articles Included

The three included studies were published between 2018 and 2022; one was a randomized control trial and two were open-label observational studies. The three studies examined changes in skin characteristics in response to the application of topical defensins to different sites: face and neck; periorbita; and hands, forearms, elbows, and knees.[19,25,26] **Table 1** shows the summary of the study design and findings from the three studies.

These studies assessed both objective and subjective outcomes. Objective structural and physiologic skin measurements were obtained with medical imaging software, LifeViz App (Quantificare, France) and DermaLab Skin Lab Combo Suite (Cortex Technology, Denmark). Quantificare is able to assess skin health (ie, evenness, pores, and oiliness) using three-dimensional image analysis and allows for individual pretreatment and posttreatment comparisons as well as for comparing individual values to a reference population that matches patients based on similar age, sex, and skin type. When comparing to the reference population, scores are provided on a range from −2 to +2 which represents the standard deviation relative to a matching population. For example, a value of +2 indicates excellent skin condition compared with a matched population. The DermaLab Combo uses probes and ultrasounds to measure dermal thickness, TEWL, elasticity, pigmentation, and hydration. In addition, skin characteristics (ie, pores, wrinkles, hyperpigmentation, erythema, scaling, and dryness) were measured subjectively with the use of the Griffiths scale by clinical investigators and with the use of consumer self-reported assessments by patients. The Griffiths scale assesses pores, superficial wrinkles, deep wrinkles, hyperpigmentation, erythema, scaling, and dryness on a scale of 0 to 4 (0—none visible, 4—severe condition).[27]

Histopathology

Histopathologic changes of the skin were assessed only in the study by Taub and colleagues, in which seven subjects (four treatment, three control) underwent punch biopsy of the postauricular skin for histopathologic analysis at 6 or 12 weeks posttreatment.[25] The treatment group showed an increase in epidermis thickness of 0.09 ± 0.02 mm compared with 0.02 ± 0.03 mm for the placebo ($P = .027$). There were no signs of inflammation in the biopsied tissue evidenced by the lack of inflammatory cells and spongiosis. In addition, there was no change in cell proliferation in the treatment and placebo groups measured by Ki-67-protein staining.

Wrinkles

After exclusion of patients with baseline Griffiths scores of 0 or 1, the study by Taub and colleagues demonstrated that 21 of 25 patients with moderate and severe conditions (Griffiths scores of 2, 3, and 4) had at least a one-grade improvement in superficial wrinkles at week 6 or week 12 compared with 6 of 25 in the placebo group ($P = .048$).[25] This finding was confirmed with Quantificare analysis which demonstrated a reduction in the number of superficial wrinkles in the treatment group. Similarly, Berens and

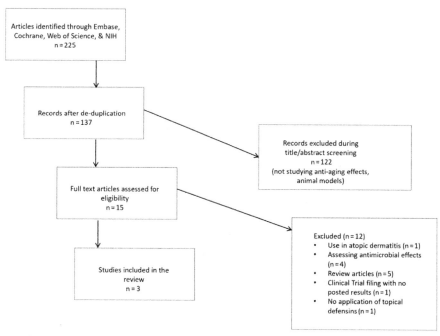

Fig. 1. PRISMA flowchart.

Table 1
Summary of the design and findings of the three studies including in the review

Study	Author, Year	Participants	Time	Intervention	Placebo	Outcomes Measured	Skin Outcome Measurement Methods	Results	Conclusion
1	Taub, 2018	44 healthy female subjects 41–71 year old	12 wk	Serum containing alpha-defensin 5 and beta-defensin 3 and other cosmetic ingredients was applied to the face, postauricular, and neck skin twice daily	Yes	Wrinkles, pores, pigmentation, thickness, elasticity, and TEWL	Histopathology (objective measures of pores, hyperpigmentation, epidermal thickness, superficial and deep wrinkles) Griffith's scale (subjective measures of pores, wrinkles, and product tolerance) SkinLab Combo Suite (objective measures of pigmentation)	Histopathology showed significant increases in all five parameters (pores, hyperpigmentation, epidermal thickness, superficial and deep wrinkles) in comparison to placebo ($P = .029$) at weeks 6 and 12; lack of inflammation and no significant proliferation of cells shown on histopathology Pore sizes significantly reduced ($P = .036$) in comparison to placebo at week 12; wrinkles significantly improved ($P = .048$) compared with placebo at weeks 6 and 12; product tolerance (erythema, scaling, and dryness) shown to improve on Griffith's scale Pigmentation significantly reduced ($P = .016$) in comparison to baseline on SkinLab analysis	The skin care regimen containing alpha and beta defensins was shown to significantly improve the appearance and structure of aging skin without irritation, dryness, and inflammation. The regimen increased epidermal thickness and reduced the appearance of pores, wrinkles, and pigmentation. In addition to these outcomes, histopathology demonstrated no significant proliferation of cells and carcinogenic markers.

#	Study	Duration	Intervention	RCT	Outcomes measured	Assessment method	Results	Conclusion
						Quantificare (objective measures of pores and oiliness)	Visible pores (skin quality) significantly improved ($P = .021$) compared with baseline, and oiliness improved ($P = .008$) compared with placebo by week 12 on Quantificare analysis	
						High-resolution 3D photography	Wrinkles significantly improved ($P = .048$); pore size, pore depth, and number of pores significantly reduced on 3D imaging	
2	Berens, 2020	6 wk	Cream containing defensins was applied to periocular region twice daily	No	Wrinkles, pores, oiliness, thickness, elasticity, hydration, and self-reported questionnaire	Patient Survey Tool (subjective changes in skin quality and aging: assessed redness, sensitivity, age spots, and wrinkles)	Subjective measures of skin quality showed a 2.1 point improvement ($P = .002$)	The use of topical eye cream containing defensins showed improvements in skin quality, including skin redness, sensitivity, age spots, and crow's feet. Objective measures showed trend toward improvement but did not reach significance.
	6 females and 2 males with periocular rhytids 37–63 year old					Quantificare (objective changes in periocular skin quality)	Quantificare imaging showed a 55% improvement in wrinkles, 12% in oiliness, 370% in pores, and no improvements in skin evenness	
						DermLab ultrasound scanner (objective changes in periocular skin quality)	DermaLab measurements showed a 28% improvement in skin thickness, 120% in elasticity, and 6% in hydration	

(continued on next page)

Danielian et al

Table 1
(continued)

Study	Author, Year	Participants	Time	Intervention	Placebo	Outcomes Measured	Skin Outcome Measurement Methods	Results	Conclusion
3	Eggerstedt, 2022	14 females with dry, photoaged, or dull skin 44–75 year old	6 wk	Hand and body cream containing defensins applied to bilateral hands, forearms, elbows, and knees twice daily	No	Skin thickness, retraction time, viscoelasticity, skin density, hydration, TEWL, and self-reported questionnaire	DermaLab Combo (objective skin structure and physiologic measurements: TEWL, elasticity, hydration, skin thickness, and density)	Dermal thickness significantly increased at all sites by 16% ($P = .002$) and collagen density by 40% ($P < .001$); elbows and above knee had the greatest improvements in skin thickness by 29% ($P = .03$) and 17% ($P = .04$) in comparison to baseline Skin density significantly increased in all sites ($P < .05$) with greatest in the hand ($P < .001$) and above knee ($P < .001$) in comparison to baseline Retraction time significantly decreased by 56% across all sites ($P < .001$) with most at the elbows by 69% ($P = .003$) and above knee at 64% ($P = .003$) in comparison to baseline	Significant improvements in skin quality, roughness, dryness, discomfort, ashiness, wrinkling, redness, age spots, and pigmentations were shown on subjective scales. Objective measures demonstrated significant improvements in skin TEWL at the elbows. Enhancements were also shown in skin hydration, elasticity, thickness, and density at all sites including hands, forearms, elbows, and knees.

	Self-reported 10-item questionnaire	

Viscoelasticity significantly improved at all sites by 50% ($P < .001$) with the greatest at the elbows by 125% ($P = .009$) and above knee by 110% ($P < .001$) in comparison to baseline

Hydration significantly improved by 31% in all sites with the most at the elbows($P < .001$), forearms ($P < .05$), and above knees ($P = .04$) in comparison to baseline

TEWL significantly improved at the elbows by 39% ($P < .02$) in comparison to baseline

Self-reported questionnaire showed significant improvements of 2.1 points in overall skin quality, roughness, dryness, discomfort, ashiness, wrinkling, redness, age spots, and pigmentations ($P < .05$) in comparison to baseline

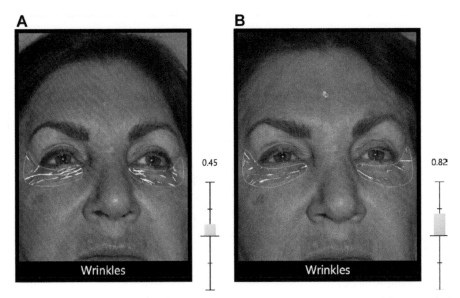

Fig. 2. Comparison of periorbital skin wrinkles pretreatment (*A*) and posttreatment (B). 3D analysis was performed on LifeViz App (Quantificare) which allows for comparison to a reference population matched for age, sex, and skin type for the parameter of "wrinkles." Scores are from −2 to +2, which indicate the standard deviation relative to the matched population with +2 being the most favorable value. This patient demonstrates a value of +0.45 pretreatment with improvement to +0.82 posttreatment. (From Berens et al., 2020 with permission.)

colleagues found a 55% improvement in periorbital wrinkles in the treatment group using Quantificare analysis; however, this finding did not reach statistical significance.[26] An example of the improvement in periorbital wrinkles following treatment is demonstrated in **Fig. 2**.

Pores

Using Quantificare analysis for the parameter "pores," Taub and colleagues demonstrated an improvement in the skin pore quality from baseline at the 12-week mark, in addition to more favorable scores compared with the matched population for the treatment group.[25] The control group did not demonstrate an improvement in pore quality. An example of the improvement in pore quality (ie, number of pores, pore size, and depth) from baseline is displayed in **Fig. 3**. Berens and colleagues found a 370% improvement in pores following treatment (statistical significance not reached).[26]

Pigmentation

In the Taub and colleagues' study, using DermaLab Combo Suite, the average pigmentation index significantly decreased from 42.09 to 40.35 ($P = .016$) after 6 weeks in the intervention group compared with no significant change in the placebo group (41.45 and 41.52 at baseline and 6 weeks, respectively).[25]

Thickness

Following exposure to defensins, increases in skin thickness on histopathology and on Dermalab Combo analysis were observed in the studies. Berens and colleagues found a 28% increase in skin thickness from pretreatment in the periorbital area (did not reach statistical significance).[26] Eggerstedt and colleagues demonstrated an increase in dermal thickness by 16% (198 μm, $P = .002$) compared with pretreatment for all body sites, with greatest improvements in the elbow (29%, 334 μm, $P = .03$) and knee (17%, 227 μm, $P = .04$).[19] Moreover, skin density (calculated as the intensity of collagen signals in the dermis on a scale of 0–100 scale) improved across all body sites tested; the greatest improvements were in the hand (47%, 11.7 points, $P < .001$), followed by above the knee area (45%, 10.1 points, $P < .001$). Taub and colleagues found a trend toward improvement (statistical significance not achieved) in dermal thickness for the treatment group (average dermal thickness was 1.49, 1.51, and 1.53 mm at baseline, 6 and 12 weeks, respectively) compared with the control group (average dermal thickness was 1.28, 1.22, and 1.26 mm at baseline, 6 and 12 weeks, respectively).[25]

Hydration

Hydration was measured with Dermalab Combo and is a measure of the water binding capacity of

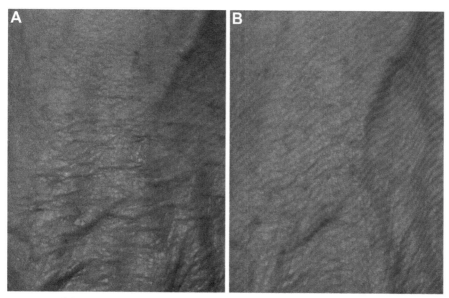

Fig. 3. Comparison of hand wrinkles before (*A*) and after treatment (*B*). Figure B demonstrates changes following 6 weeks of application of a topical defensin to the hand. (Figure from Eggerstedt et al., 2022 with permission.)

the stratus corneum. Periorbital skin demonstrated a 6% improvement in hydration (not statistically significant).[26] There was an average 31% increase in skin hydration among all body sites (elbow, hands, forearm, and above the knee) with the elbow (99% increase, 53.5 μS, $P < .001$) and above knee regions (28%, 22.4 μS, $P = .04$) demonstrating the largest improvements.[19]

Transepidermal Water Loss

Dermalab Combo was used to measure TEWL defined as the evaporation rate of water through the outer layer of the epidermis. Taub and colleagues demonstrated a trend toward improvement in TEWL score following treatment ($P>.05$).[25] The average TEWL in the treatment group decreased from 32.54 mg/cm²/h at baseline to 11.24 mg/cm²/h at 6 weeks and to 15.02 mg/cm²/h at 12 weeks. In contrast, the control group did not demonstrate an improvement in TEWL: 19.03 mg/cm²/h, 15.68 mg/cm²/h, and 24.20 mg/cm²/h at baseline, 6 and 12 weeks, respectively. Similarly, Eggerstedt and colleagues also found improvements following treatment: TEWL significantly improved at the elbow by 39% (−4.1 g/m²/h, $P = .02$) and trended toward improvement in the hand (19%, −3.2 g/m²/h, $P = .2$).[19]

Self-Reported

Subjective measures of skin were reported in two of the studies aiming to assess patients' perception of improvement in skin quality by rating skin characteristics pretreatment and posttreatment

(scale 1–7). For the periorbital region, patients reported an average 2.1 point improvement in overall skin quality compared with pretreatment($P = .002$), with greatest improvements in sensitivity to weather (3.3 points), age spots (2.8 points), crow's feet (2.9 points) (P-values not provided).[26] Similarly, patients who applied the cream to body sites (hands, elbow, forearms, and knees) reported an average 2.1 point improvement ($P<.001$) in the overall skin quality, with improvements in skin roughness (1.6 points), dryness (2.6 points), discomfort (1.6 points), ashiness (2.2 points), wrinkling (2.0 points), redness (1.4 points), age spots (1.6 points), and pigmentation (1.8 points) (P-values < 0.05).[19] Moreover, patient satisfaction with the cream was high with 86% reporting they would recommend the cream to a friend.[19]

Tolerance

Although there were no tolerance issues present in the studies by Taub and colleagues and Berens and colleagues, 2 out of 22 patients in the Eggerstedt and colleagues study experienced skin sensitivity and discontinued the use of cream. Product tolerance assessed with a consumer survey did note improvements in facial skin discomfort during the day, sensitivity to cold weather, redness, and tingling/burning/stinging with application of the topical.[25]

Stem Cell Proliferation

One important concern with stimulating stem cells with growth factors is the risk of promoting carcinogenesis. To assess this, Taub and colleagues demonstrated no increase in the number of proliferating cells, measured with expression levels of Ki-67, a DNA-binding nuclear protein present in dividing cells.[25]

DISCUSSION

Aging skin is characterized by increases in wrinkles, pigmentation, skin water loss and moisture, and reductions in elasticity. Commonly used commercial products aimed at targeting the aging phenotypes include topical growth factors, retinols, and chemical peels that induce new skin growth.[28] Topicals are not without undesirable effects and can lead to cellular senescence, uncontrolled replication, and inflammatory response. As the science of antiaging advances, new ingredients emerge in the market.[29,30] Thus, this systematic review aimed to assess a new ingredient, defensins, and its potential to target aging skin. Three studies meeting inclusion criteria were identified which evaluated the antiaging effects of topical defensins on skin.

Alpha- and beta-defensins are AMPs that are naturally released by the skin in response to skin injury. Once released, defensins activate LGR6+ multipotent stem cells, which play an integral role in epidermal growth given their ability to differentiate into all lineages of skin.[21,31] The role of LGR6+ stem cells in wound healing also provides insight into its role in epidermal homeostasis. LGR6+ stem cells are crucial in initiating the reepithelialization process and impairing their contribution significantly delays wound healing.[32] A study by Lough and colleagues, in which LGR6+ stem cells were transplanted into wound beds in mice, showed enhanced wound healing and augmentation of vascular endothelial growth factor and platelet-derived growth factor pathways when compared with controls.[22] Alpha- and beta-defensin peptides also contain pro-immunity, antibacterial, and antitumor effects.[21,33–36] Owing to these characteristics of skin rejuvenation, defensins have garnered attention as agents to improve skin composition.

One of the studies included in this review was by Taub and colleagues which assessed the antiaging effects of defensins by applying α-defensin 5 and β-defensin 3 to the face, postauricular area, and neck.[25] The study demonstrated that the use of defensins improved the structure of aging skin without causing skin irritation, dryness, or inflammation. The effectiveness of the regimen was assessed using a range of clinical, histopathologic, immunohistochemical, photographic, and ultrasound evaluation methods. Histopathology demonstrated improvements in epidermal thickness, decrease in pores, hyperpigmentation,

superficial and deep wrinkles without inflammatory changes. Moreover, objective analysis with 3D imaging, Quantificare, SkinLab, and the Griffiths scale showed improvements in wrinkles, pores, pigmentation, evenness of skin surface, and oiliness by week 12. An important finding of this study was the lack of excessive cell proliferation as measured by Ki-67 immunohistochemistry which is a concern when stem cells proliferation is part of the mechanism of action.

The study by Berens and colleagues revealed both subjective and objective improvements in the periocular skin quality following application of topical defensins.[26] Subjectively, skin redness, sensitivity, age spots, and crow's feet wrinkles had improvements after 6 weeks use of the defensin topicals. Objectively, measures with Quantificare analysis demonstrated improvements in skin wrinkles, oiliness, and pores, and Dermalab ultrasound analysis showed improvements in skin thickness, elasticity, and hydration. Although improvements in both objective and subjective measures were realized, only subjective measures of skin quality reached statistical significance in this study.

The third study assessed the changes in skin composition of the body including the hands, forearms, elbows, and knees using DermaLab analysis and subjective measures.[19] After 6 weeks of defensin topical use, significant improvements were revealed in dermal thickness at the knee and elbow, and improvements in collagen density, skin elasticity, and skin density at all sites using. Moisture content improved at the elbows, forearms, and above knee areas, whereas TEWL significantly improved at the elbows. Moreover, subjective measures showed significant improvements in overall skin quality roughness, dryness, discomfort, ashiness, wrinkling, redness, age spots, and pigmentation of skin after 6 weeks of use. Although most of the measured body sites demonstrated improvements, the back of the hand did not demonstrate measurable improvements. The authors proposed that this may be due to hands being washed more frequently than other body surfaces and as a result, reducing exposure time to the topical.

Limitations and Future Studies

The major limitation of this study is the small number of studies in the literature studying the effects of topical defensins on skin composition. After literature review, only three studies were identified which were heterogeneous in the face and body sites tested. Taub and colleagues measured the effects in the face and neck region, Berens and colleagues in the periocular regions, and Eggerstedt and colleagues on the body (eg, hands, forearms, elbows, and knees).[19,25,26] Thus, more studies are required to test the effects of topical defensins at the same anatomic sites to provide more robust sample sizes. Moreover, the studies differed in study cohorts, whereas two studies included only female participants,[19,25] one had both female and male participants.[26] Future studies should aim to incorporate both male and female participants and include a larger cohort with diverse ethnic backgrounds to reduce heterogeneity among the studies. Furthermore, future research may reduce bias by including a blinded control group to improve validity of the study. Last, although overall patient tolerance to the topical defensins seems to be great, there were two patients in the study by Eggerstedt and colleagues that withdrew from the study due to sensitivity issues. Thus, investigations into circumstances that lead to sensitivity to defensin topicals should be elucidated with further research. Similarly, it would be interesting to compare defensins to commonly used topicals on the market, such as retinols which may be characterized by side effects such as retinoid dermatitis[37] to assess differences in tolerability and skin composition outcomes.

SUMMARY

Overall, these studies suggest topical defensins are effective in improving the skin composition of the face, eyes, and other body sites. Improvements in skin elasticity, skin moisture content, TEWL, pigmentation, pores, and wrinkles were demonstrated in all three studies without major side effects. However, research on the antiaging effects of topical defensins is in the early stages and larger studies will be needed to generalize the results.

CLINICS CARE POINTS

- Alpha- and beta-defensins are antimicrobial peptides that stimulate LGR6+ stem cells, which sit above the hair follicle bulge in the basal epidermal layer of the skin.
- This review of the literature demonstrates improvements in skin elasticity, skin moisture content, transepidermal water loss, pigmentation, pores, and wrinkles of the face and body can be achieved with the application of topical defensins.
- Although defensins stimulate stem cells, there is no evidence of excessive cell proliferation on histopathologic analysis to indicate a carcinogenic potential.

- Topical defensins are tolerated well by patients with only two patients from the three studies reporting skin sensitivity and discontinuing its use.
- Topical defensins can play a role in the skin care routine of patients aiming to target antiaging.

ETHICS APPROVAL AND CONSENT TO PARTICIPATE

This review did not require IRB approval as it did not constitute human subject research.

DISCLOSURE STATEMENT

The authors have no financial interests to disclose. No funding was received for this work.

AUTHORS' CONTRIBUTIONS

R.P.R. Kerr: design, conduct, analysis, presentation; A. Danielian: design, conduct, analysis, presentation; M. Danielian: design, conduct, analysis; P.S. Han: analysis, presentation; M.Y. Cheng: analysis, presentation.

REFERENCES

1. Ahmed IA, Mikail MA, Zamakshshari N, et al. Natural anti-aging skincare: role and potential. Biogerontology 2020;21(3):293–310.
2. Verschoore M, Nielson M. The Rationale of Anti-Aging Cosmetic Ingredients. J Drugs Dermatol JDD 2017;16(6):s94–7.
3. Zachary CM, Wang JV, Saedi N. Resveratrol as a Skincare Ingredient: Current Evidence and the Future Potential. Skinmed 2021;19(6):414–6.
4. Costa EF, Magalhães WV, Di Stasi LC. Recent Advances in Herbal-Derived Products with Skin Anti-Aging Properties and Cosmetic Applications. Molecules 2022;27(21):7518.
5. Bhat BB, Kamath PP, Chatterjee S, et al. Recent Updates on Nanocosmeceutical Skin Care and Anti-Aging Products. Curr Pharm Des 2022;28(15):1258–71.
6. Scientific Committee of Consumer Safety - SCCS. Electronic address: SANTE-C2-SCCS@ec.europa.eu, Rousselle C. Opinion of the Scientific Committee on Consumer Safety (SCCS) - Final version of the Opinion on Vitamin A (retinol, retinyl acetate and retinyl palmitate) in cosmetic products. Regul Toxicol Pharmacol RTP 2017;84:102–4.
7. Dhaliwal S, Rybak I, Ellis SR, et al. Prospective, randomized, double-blind assessment of topical bakuchiol and retinol for facial photoageing. Br J Dermatol 2019;180(2):289–96.

8. Till JE, McCulloch EA. A Direct Measurement of the Radiation Sensitivity of Normal Mouse Bone Marrow Cells. Radiat Res 2012;178(2):AV3–7.

9. Nair N, Gongora E. Stem cell therapy in heart failure: Where do we stand today? Biochim Biophys Acta Mol Basis Dis 2020;1866(4):165489.

10. Khalid K, Padda J, Wijeratne Fernando R, et al. Stem Cell Therapy and Its Significance in HIV Infection. Cureus 2021;13(8):e17507.

11. Passweg JR, Baldomero H, Bader P, et al. Hematopoietic stem cell transplantation in Europe 2014: more than 40 000 transplants annually. Bone Marrow Transplant 2016;51(6):786–92.

12. Yamazaki K, Kawabori M, Seki T, et al. Clinical Trials of Stem Cell Treatment for Spinal Cord Injury. Int J Mol Sci 2020;21(11):3994.

13. Taub AF, Pham K. Stem Cells in Dermatology and Anti-aging Care of the Skin. Facial Plast Surg Clin N Am 2018;26(4):425–37.

14. Ho CY, Dreesen O. Faces of cellular senescence in skin aging. Mech Ageing Dev 2021;198:111525.

15. Trautinger F. Mechanisms of photodamage of the skin and its functional consequences for skin ageing: Photodamage and skin ageing. Clin Exp Dermatol 2001;26(7):573–7.

16. Yaar M, Gilchrest BA. Skin aging. Clin Geriatr Med 2001;17(4):617–30.

17. Bonté F, Girard D, Archambault JC, et al. Skin Changes During Ageing. In: Harris JR, Korolchuk VI, editors. Biochemistry and cell biology of ageing: Part II clinical science. Vol 91. Subcellular biochemistry. Springer Singapore; 2019. p. 249–80. https://doi.org/10.1007/978-981-13-3681-2_10.

18. Makrantonaki E, Zouboulis CC. Molecular Mechanisms of Skin Aging: State of the Art. Ann N Y Acad Sci 2007;1119(1):40–50.

19. Eggerstedt M, Torres-Maldonado S, Danielian A, et al. Impact of defensins-containing body cream on skin composition. J Cosmet Dermatol 2023;22(2):620–7.

20. Gao X, Ding J, Liao C, et al. Defensins: The natural peptide antibiotic. Adv Drug Deliv Rev 2021;179:114008.

21. Snippert HJ, Haegebarth A, Kasper M, et al. Lgr6 Marks Stem Cells in the Hair Follicle That Generate All Cell Lineages of the Skin. Science 2010;327(5971):1385–9.

22. Lough DM, Yang M, Blum A, et al. Transplantation of the LGR6+ Epithelial Stem Cell into Full-Thickness Cutaneous Wounds Results in Enhanced Healing, Nascent Hair Follicle Development, and Augmentation of Angiogenic Analytes. Plast Reconstr Surg 2014;133(3):579–90.

23. Lough D, Dai H, Yang M, et al. Stimulation of the Follicular Bulge LGR5+ and LGR6+ Stem Cells with the Gut-Derived Human Alpha Defensin 5 Results in Decreased Bacterial Presence, Enhanced Wound Healing, and Hair Growth from Tissues Devoid of Adnexal Structures. Plast Reconstr Surg 2013;132(5):1159–71.

24. Niyonsaba F, Ogawa H. Protective roles of the skin against infection: Implication of naturally occurring human antimicrobial agents β-defensins, cathelicidin LL-37 and lysozyme. J Dermatol Sci 2005;40(3):157–68.

25. Taub A, Bucay V, Keller G, et al. Multi-Center, Double-Blind, Vehicle-Controlled Clinical Trial of an Alpha and Beta Defensin-Containing Anti-Aging Skin Care Regimen With Clinical, Histopathologic, Immunohistochemical, Photographic, and Ultrasound Evaluation. J Drugs Dermatol JDD 2018;17(4):426–41.

26. Berens AM, Ghazizadeh S. Effect of defensins-containing eye cream on periocular rhytids and skin quality. J Cosmet Dermatol 2020;19(8):2000–5.

27. Griffiths CE, Wang TS, Hamilton TA, et al. A photonumeric scale for the assessment of cutaneous photodamage. Arch Dermatol 1992;128(3):347–51.

28. Shao Y, He T, Fisher GJ, et al. Molecular basis of retinol anti-ageing properties in naturally aged human skin in vivo. Int J Cosmet Sci 2017;39(1):56–65.

29. Berry K, Hallock K, Lam C. Photoaging and Topical Rejuvenation. Facial Plast Surg Clin N Am 2022;30(3):291–300.

30. Gorouhi F, Maibach HI. Role of topical peptides in preventing or treating aged skin. Int J Cosmet Sci 2009;31(5):327–45.

31. Xue Y, Lyu C, Taylor A, et al. Mechanical tension mobilizes Lgr6+ epidermal stem cells to drive skin growth. Sci Adv 2022;8(17):eabl8698.

32. Huang S, Kuri P, Aubert Y, et al. Lgr6 marks epidermal stem cells with a nerve-dependent role in wound re-epithelialization. Cell Stem Cell 2021;28(9):1582–96.e6.

33. Kudryashova E, Quintyn R, Seveau S, et al. Human Defensins Facilitate Local Unfolding of Thermodynamically Unstable Regions of Bacterial Protein Toxins. Immunity 2014;41(5):709–21.

34. Hanaoka Y, Yamaguchi Y, Yamamoto H, et al. In Vitro and In Vivo Anticancer Activity of Human β-Defensin-3 and Its Mouse Homolog. Anticancer Res 2016;36(11):5999–6004.

35. Lichtenstein A, Ganz T, Selsted ME, et al. In vitro tumor cell cytolysis mediated by peptide defensins of human and rabbit granulocytes. Blood 1986;68(6):1407–10.

36. Semple F, Dorin JR. β-Defensins: Multifunctional Modulators of Infection, Inflammation and More? J Innate Immun 2012;4(4):337–48.

37. Culp L, Tuchayi SM, Alinia H, et al. Tolerability of topical retinoids: Are there clinically meaningful differences among topical retinoids? J Cutan Med Surg 2015;19(6).

Holistic Approach for Noninvasive Facial Rejuvenation by Simultaneous Use of High Intensity Focused Electrical Stimulation and Synchronized Radiofrequency
A Review of Treatment Effects Underlined by Understanding of Facial Anatomy

Suneel Chilukuri, MD

KEYWORDS

• Face • Fillers • High intensity focused electrical stimulation • Radiofrequency • Neuromodulators
• Noninvasive

KEY POINTS

- Facial aging is a continuous process resulting from age-related changes in all structures present in the face. Such complex anatomy needs to be considered when it comes to noninvasive treatments for improving facial appearance. The facial muscles especially should be seen within their connective tissue environment and addressed accordingly.
- Novel HIFES and Synchronized RF technology was developed to target facial layers in synergy. Its effects show that it is a viable option for noninvasive face lifting and wrinkle reduction.
- It has been documented that HIFES and Synchronized RF does not interfere with the effects of neuromodulators or dermal fillers and can be safely and effectively used in patients injected with either of them, to deliver satisfactory improvement of overall facial appearance.

INTRODUCTION

Facial aging is a continuous process resulting from age-related changes in all structures present in the face: skin, fat, muscle, fascia, and bone.[1,2] Age-related changes of all facial soft tissues start at different decades and progress at various paces, which vary between individuals of different gender and ethnicity. All changes together result in reduced support for the bone-overlying soft tissues, which then follow the effect of gravity. Thus, a loss of structural support owing to volume depletion and changes to the facial muscles and their connective tissue framework results in increased soft tissue laxity.

The Role of Facial Muscles and Fascia Framework in Aesthetic Appearance

Facial muscles have been found to age through the process of sarcopenia, which manifests as a loss of muscle mass and volume, similar to skeletal muscles.[3] Because the facial muscles are interconnected via the fascial system and the

Refresh Dermatology, 5427 Bissonnet Street #500, Houston, TX 77081, USA
E-mail address: chilukuri@refreshdermatology.com

Facial Plast Surg Clin N Am 31 (2023) 547–555
https://doi.org/10.1016/j.fsc.2023.06.006
1064-7406/23/© 2023 Elsevier Inc. All rights reserved.

overlying skin, weakening of these muscles may result in a visible descent of the tissue as we age (**Fig. 1**). The weaker the facial muscles are, and the lower the resting muscle tone is, the higher that muscle effort is needed to avoid sagging and to hold the overlying tissues in place. When too weak, they become unable to hold the tissue, resulting in eyebrow drop or cheek sagging. When the resting muscle tone is increased, the muscles are then able to hold the overlying tissue in place without dropping and without the need to stay contracted.

Specifically, the muscles in the cheek are interconnected by the midfacial superficial musculoaponeurotic system (SMAS).[4] Weakening of the cheek muscles, especially the zygomaticus muscles, allows for the hypothesis that as we age, the resulting facial muscle weakness can promote midfacial soft tissue descent, resulting in the increased severity of the nasolabial fold, formation of jowls, and loss of jawline contour.[5] Targeting these muscles and their surrounding connective tissue architecture might allow for midfacial soft tissue repositioning. Also, the same muscle weakening could be expected for the frontalis muscle owing to aging or long-term use of neurotoxins. The frontalis muscle is mainly responsible for eyebrow movements. Its connection with the skin is ensured via the suprafrontalis fascia (located superficial to the frontalis muscle) and the subfrontalis fascia (located deep below the frontalis muscle). Aging of the forehead structures may result in eyebrow ptosis[6] and heaviness, which along with skin aging, may lead to laxity and wrinkle formation in the region.

In contrast to skeletal muscles, the facial muscles are embedded in a connective tissue framework that interconnects all tissues from bone to skin. Interestingly, they are connected directly to the brain via the cranial nerves and are responsive to emotional input and the limbic system. Emotional states affect facial contours via resting tone of the muscles and the SMAS. Therefore, the facial muscles need to be seen within their connective tissue environment and addressed accordingly. Assuming that facial muscles affect skin movement alone without the support of a connective tissue environment creates an incomplete picture of facial muscle anatomy.

Treatment Alternatives

Repositioning and restructuring the facial tissues and layers is the aim of aesthetic procedures via surgical and nonsurgical means.[1,2] Among noninvasive aesthetic procedures, radiofrequency (RF) is considered the gold standard for facial skin treatment. The effect of RF on the skin tissue is based on dermal heating, which leads to structural changes within the skin and the overall improvement in skin quality.[7] However, these skin heating procedures focus solely on improving skin quality and textural improvement, but not the overall facial appearance, which is also influenced by the facial volume and density of the underlying structures, including the fascial system, facial ligaments, and facial muscles. Therefore, the extent of facial laxity is a composite effect of all implicated structures of which the facial muscles and their interconnection with the skin play a fundamental role.[8]

The most frequently performed nonsurgical treatment to date is the administration of soft tissue fillers, which helps to restore facial volume. However, soft tissue fillers only cover the aging symptoms and do not affect facial muscles, which play a crucial role in natural skin mobility.[9] When it comes to muscles, the application of neurotoxins is yet another popular solution, although its primary effects are also limited to one tissue only. Currently, the only way to reliably alter facial muscles is through a surgical lift procedure, where the skin and fat tissues are separated from the muscle, and the muscles are then repositioned.[10]

Overall, the combination of age-related facial changes results in an alteration of the facial shape, which cannot be improved by targeting one type of tissue alone. Therefore, more profound treatment algorithms need to be applied to address age-related facial changes.[11] This may include addressing deeper fascial and muscle layers

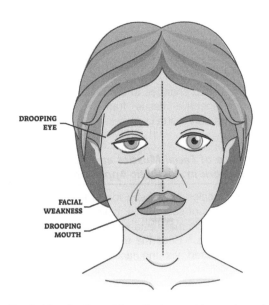

DROOPING EYE

FACIAL WEAKNESS

DROOPING MOUTH

Fig. 1. Visualization of the effect caused by weakened facial muscles on the left in comparison to healthy muscles on the right.

together, as they have the ability to promote facial repositioning.

Recently, HIFES technology synchronized with RF heating has been introduced with the EMFACE (BTL Industries Ltd, Boston, MA, USA) device, to target the facial muscles and their connective tissue frameworks for lifting and tightening of the facial contours. HIFES technology induces electrical fields to contract facial muscles selectively. These delicate facial muscles are crucial for supporting the facial soft tissues and play a structural role in a more youthful appearance. While the HIFES targets the muscle and overlying fascia tissue, the Synchronized RF heating induces structural changes to the dermal and subdermal architecture. This approach can ultimately result in an improved appearance through changes in all facial tissue layers.

TARGETING FACIAL TISSUES BY NONINVASIVE HIFES AND SYNCHRONIZED RADIOFREQUENCY TECHNOLOGIES
Mechanics of HIFES for Facial Muscle Stimulation

HIFES technology was specifically designed to selectively induce supramaximal contractions of small delicate muscles in the face, namely the frontalis muscle on the forehead and zygomaticus major muscles, zygomaticus minor muscles and risorius muscles on the cheeks (**Fig. 2**). The technology generates strong electrical fields, delivered by its specifically designed applicators, that affect the underlying neuronal and muscle tissue. These electrical fields depolarize the membrane of the motor neurons that innervate the muscle. When the motor neurons are depolarized, a signal is

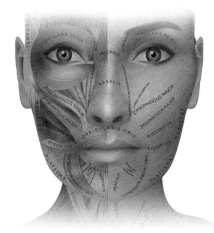

Fig. 2. The cheek muscles stimulated by HIFES technology: zygomaticus major and minor muscles and risorius muscle.

created that travels along the neuron, all the way to the neuromuscular junction—the place where the motor neuron is connected to the muscle. These signals overcome the barrier of the neuromuscular junction and progress to the muscle, which is thus forced to contract. This process bypasses the voluntary intention of the brain, inducing a forced contraction through electrical stimulation.

The HIFES stimuli repeat with such frequency that the facial muscles are not allowed to relax in between the individual signals. As the muscle cannot relax, with additional stimuli, it is forced to contract even further, which continuously builds up the contraction power with every additional signal. The appropriate selection of these 2 factors (electrical field strength and frequency) results in the so-called supramaximal contraction. Although it is poorly understood how and to what extent the facial muscles adapt to external stimuli, research studies conducted in skeletal muscles have revealed that heat shock proteins (HSP) and satellite cells (SCs) may be activated by intense muscle exercise as a response to the applied stimuli.[12] HSPs are the signaling molecules playing a crucial role in muscle remodeling through the promotion of muscle protein synthesis.[13] SCs are muscle-derived stem cells responsible for myofiber development and renewal.[14] In a resting state, the SCs remain quiescent, ready to be activated, and provide differentiation to create new myonuclei to existing muscle fibers or generate new muscle fibers. Together, HSP and SC activation can support muscle microprotein structure alterations. In a healthy muscle this may lead to densification of the muscle tissue and to overall improvement of the muscle quality. In atrophied muscle, the muscle structure alteration may lead to hypertrophic response reversing the atrophy. However, it is not only the muscle reacting to the signaling molecules. It has also been documented that the fascial layer remodels itself in response to heat and mechanical stimuli.[15] Nonetheless, the future studies will need to identify similarities between skeletal and facial muscles or provide conclusive evidence that facial muscles behave similarly or differently when targeted by external stimuli.

The Role of Synchronized Radiofrequency Heating on Facial Muscles and Framework

Simultaneously with the HIFES stimulation, the Synchronized RF that heats the facial tissue is delivered. Such stimuli affect the connective tissue framework and the facial muscle unit with consecutive adaptive changes to the overlying facial soft tissues. According to previous studies on skeletal muscles,[13,16] HSPs can also be activated by heat within the range of 40°C. Together with the muscular contractions, the heat thus may further increase the levels of released HSP,[17] although this effect has been shown in abdominal muscle[18] or gluteal muscle.[19] A recent study by Kinney and colleagues[20] measured the facial muscle temperature during the treatment with HIFES and RF and showed that the temperatures in the targeted muscle tissues reached up to 40°C, indicating that a similar effect could also be seen in the facial muscles during the simultaneous treatment.

Furthermore, the primary effect of Synchronized RF heating on the subdermal tissues can be seen in the fascial framework. The fascial framework primarily consists of collagen and elastin, which are known to be heat responsive. Therefore, heating to adequate temperatures may induce remodeling of collagen and elastin within the fascial framework, leading to increased elasticity and tightness of the fascial web.[15]

The Role of Synchronized Radiofrequency Heating on Skin Tissue Rejuvenation

The same effect for the fascia can also be seen in the skin tissue. Regarding skin, fine lines and wrinkles accompanied by loss of skin volume are usually the first indicators of skin aging, a normal physiologic process influenced by genetic and hormonal changes with contribution of external factors.[21] During the skin aging process, the dermal blood vessel structure is disrupted, and in turn, the dermis is not supplied with nutrition and oxygen, thus slowing cellular regeneration.

The major building blocks of the skin are collagen and elastin fibers, which are responsible for skin elasticity and firmness. During the aging process, collagen and elastin synthesis decreases, and collagen bundles lose their extensible configuration and become fragmented. The elastin fiber network is degraded, leading to the loss of structural integrity of microfibrils. As the extracellular matrix is degraded, skin thickness is also reduced. It is estimated that adult skin loses 1% of overall collagen content annually.[22]

The EMFACE device uses a novel Synchronized RF electrode that allows the simultaneous application of an RF field together with HIFES. As the RF current flows through the tissue, a portion of the RF energy is absorbed, transforming the energy into heat and the desired thermal effect. During the 20-minute treatment, the skin tissue is heated to 40°C to 42°C. This therapeutic temperature range is reached within the first 2 minutes of the treatment, as documented by the thermal probe

measurements.[23] The level of RF energy absorption in the tissue depends on the RF frequency and tissue impedance, among other factors. Because the skin, muscle, and fat tissues have different impedances,[24] it is possible to selectively target the energy and achieve the thermal effect in the desired tissues.

When the therapeutic temperature is reached in the skin tissue for the desired time period, the hydrogen bonds tying the collagen fibers together begin to unwind, and collagen denaturation occurs. However, the above-mentioned temperatures do not lead to permanent damage. As the thermal effect dissipates, the bonds begin to renew, and the skin's architecture is changed to a more youthful level. After repeating this process during multiple treatments, the structure of older collagen and elastin fibers is changed, similar to newly formed collagen and elastin fibers.[25] This thermal effect is also accompanied by a heat-induced wound-healing response and increased fibroblast activity. Fibroblasts are the dermal cells responsible for producing new collagen and elastin fibers. As we age, their activity decreases to a level equivalent to an overall "net loss" of fibers. This means that the amount of newly formed fibers does not exceed the number of fibers being degraded, which accelerates the appearance of skin aging. Nevertheless, studies have shown that heat stress increases fibroblast activity, leading to an increased synthesis of collagen and elastin–neocollagenesis and neoelastinogenesis.[25] Overall, synchronized RF heating supports the skin to regain its volume, elasticity, and a more youthful appearance by restoring the collagen and elastin fiber structure and enhancing the synthesis of new collagen fibers.

CLINICAL EFFECTS OF HIFES AND SYNCHRONIZED RADIOFREQUENCY ON FACIAL TISSUES

Because of the unique design and energy delivery, HIFES does not induce the stimulation of the depressors because it could potentially lead to a worsening of rhytides. The forehead application targets the frontalis muscle (brow elevator) and corresponding fascias while avoiding the depressors in the glabella. Restoring the tonus of the frontalis muscle and tightening the fascias in combination with the skin remodeling thus lead to reduced horizontal forehead lines, brow elevation, and skin texture improvement. The cheek application primarily targets the more superficial muscles of the cheeks (zygomaticus major/minor and risorius), which are all interconnected elevating units. In contrast, other deeper muscles, such as the masseter muscle, are unaffected. Stimulation of these superficial muscles leads to an elevation of the entire cheek, increasing the midfacial volume and improving the nasolabial fold. Increasing the pull of these elevators further leads to a repositioning not only of the midface but also of the lower facial soft tissues. The resulting clinical effect is a reduction in jowls and an increase in jawline contouring. Furthermore, the combined effect of HIFES with Synchronized RF manifests as an overall textural improvement of the skin.

Clinical studies focusing on structural changes after HIFES and RF demonstrated a prominent skin remodeling effect. These studies found that collagen increase ranged between 26% and 27%, and elastin increase ranged between 110% and 129% 2 to 3 months following the procedure.[23,26] Research[27] investigating changes in skin texture and facial appearance reported a 37% wrinkle reduction and a 25% skin evenness improvement 3 months after the procedure. The processes induced in muscle tissue led to structural remodeling of the targeted muscles, which has been documented by Kinney and colleagues,[20] showing a 19% increase in muscle density and a 21% increase in the number of myonuclei. These results were coupled with reduced fibrotic and fat infiltration within the muscle tissue at 2 months after the procedure (**Fig. 3**).

The structural changes do manifest as increased resting muscular tone, which is necessary for maintaining the lifted facial appearance. The weaker the facial muscles are, the higher the muscle effort that is needed to avoid sagging and to hold the overlying tissues in place. When too weak, they become unable to hold the tissue, resulting in, for example, eyebrow drop or cheek sagging.[2] Recently, HIFES and RF was found to increase the muscle tone by 30%,[28] which was then shown to lead to an overall lifting effect by 23%.[29] Aside from multiple clinical studies using various evaluation methods, the results of the procedure are supported by a high patient satisfaction rate of 91%.[29]

APPLICATION OF HIFES AND SYNCHRONIZED RADIOFREQUENCY THERAPY WITH CURRENTLY USED PROCEDURES FOR IMPROVEMENT OF FACIAL APPEARANCE
HIFES Effects on Neurotoxin-Blocked Muscles

Neuromodulators in aesthetic medicine, such as Botox, Dysport, Xeomin, or Jeuveau, have become some of the most frequently sought nonsurgical aesthetic procedures with type A botulinum–based neurotoxins having a myriad of clinical indications. They are most frequently used to treat dynamic facial rhytides[30] involving the glabella, frontalis, and periocular regions. Botulinum neurotoxins block neurotransmitter release (Acetylcholine; Ach) in the synaptic neuromuscular junction and block voluntary muscle contraction. With blocked contractions, wrinkle formation is prevented, as the overlying skin is not being repetitively folded during daily activities and thus aids in maintaining a more youthful skin appearance.

Botulinum-based neurotoxin affects the process of muscular contraction at the level of neuromuscular junction. When applied, it works as a protease and prevents the fusion of the vesicles with the presynaptic membrane.[31] Without this fusion, the Ach

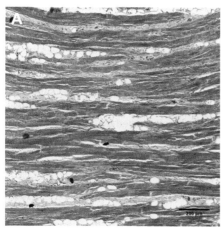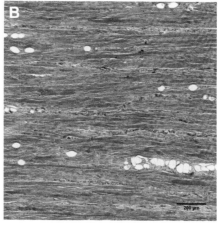

Fig. 3. Histologic images of muscle tissues before (*A*) and 2 months after (*B*) the treatment with the HIFES and RF. Red represents muscle tissue; green represents intersected collagen fibers, and white rounded cells are adipocytes.

cannot be released into the neuromuscular junction and trigger the muscle contraction. It is a chemical denervation that causes partial paralysis of the innervated muscle. However, such paralysis is not causing any damage to the nerve or the neuromuscular junction and is not permanent.[32]

Studies have shown it is possible to stimulate even the botulinum-paralyzed muscles.[33,34] However, it is not entirely clear how such stimulation overcomes the barrier made by the botulinum neurotoxin. Upon the application of botulinum toxin, the membrane of the presynaptic neuron should be practically impermeable to Ach molecules owing to its size as the fusion of vesicles and presynaptic membrane ("quantal release") is blocked. Nevertheless, clinical trials are showing that externally it is possible to overcome this barrier, and although the mechanism of how this happens is not entirely clear, several hypotheses were proposed to explain such mechanism, particularly the nonquantal Ach release[35] and direct stimulation of postsynaptic membrane.[36]

Research has shown that a nonquantal release of small amounts of Ach into the synapse still occurs, even in botulinum toxin denervated muscle. However, during voluntary contractions, the amount of the Ach is not sufficient to cause depolarization, and the muscles thus remain relaxed. By applying an external high-frequency electrical field that surpasses the frequency of brain signals, the activity of the high-affinity choline transporter could be elevated, leading to exaggerated nonquantal release of Ach in amounts sufficient enough to cause muscle depolarization and contraction. In addition, an insufficient long-term concentration of Ach in the synapse, owing to the application of botulinum toxin, can lead to an increased expression of n-acetylcholine receptor on the postsynaptic membrane and, therefore, also to an increase in the sensitivity of the muscle to Ach.[37] A lower amount of Ach would thus be needed to induce such depolarization.

On the other hand, the conclusions regarding the direct muscle stimulation are based on studies performed on skeletal muscles only. Facial muscles are of significantly different proportions and are much more superficially located in low depths. All this may influence the response. As the facial muscles are more delicate, lower intensity of stimulus may suffice to irritate the muscle membrane. Because the thickness of some facial muscles may be as small as 0.5 mm,[38] it may be possible that such stimulation is able to recruit enough muscle fibers to induce contraction of the entire muscle.

Regardless of the mechanism, HIFES technology is seemingly able to stimulate botulinum neurotoxin–blocked muscles in order to prevent risk of muscle atrophy. HIFES stimulates blocked facial muscle even though it is not possible voluntarily. Recent findings[39] showed that during the EMFACE treatment the botulinum-denervated muscles are being contracted, and what is most important, it does not interfere with the effect of botulinum toxin itself. No negative effects of the HIFES and RF procedure on the efficacy of the botulinum toxin were found.

Synchronized Radiofrequency and Dermal Fillers Treatment

Injection of dermatologic fillers is one of the most common procedures that is used in aesthetic medicine for rejuvenation of the face. These gellike substances are used for the treatment of wrinkles by injecting filler beneath the skin so it restores lost volume and more contour to the face. Fillers can be divided into 2 categories. First, the biodegradable fillers that are not permanent and can last up to 12 months, losing their effectiveness with time and eventually being metabolized. Fillers that are currently available stimulate neocollagenesis, so the effect persists longer to some extent.[40] Such dermal fillers that are currently used and approved by the Food and Drug Administration (FDA) are hyaluronic acid, calcium hydroxylapatite, and poly-L-lactic acid. The second group of nonbiodegradable fillers are long-term solutions for wrinkles, but there is a much bigger risk of complications. There are only 2 nonbiodegradable fillers approved by the FDA: polymethylmethacrylate microspheres and liquid injectable silicone (LIS), but LIS was approved only for intraocular use.[41]

Concerns have been voiced among patients and practitioners regarding RF treatments in that dermal filler would break down if they underwent RF treatment, or even worse, that the patient's skin would get damaged under RF applicators. Nevertheless, there exists plenty of evidence in the literature about safety of RF treatment over the area injected with dermal fillers.[42–44] In addition, there even exist devices that are using RF energy during dermal filler injection. In study by Kim and colleagues,[45] it was found that using RF during filler injection is a safe and effective method to treat especially mobile areas like the nasolabial fold. Overall, the findings prove that increasing the temperature of the tissue above normal levels is safe for the filler's stability. Depending on the system used, RF devices for noninvasive skin treatments elevate the tissue temperature no more than 65°C. On the other hand, the current dermal fillers are usually autoclaved, and therefore, bear considerable thermal stability. For instance, hyaluronic acid fillers are usually sterilized at a temperature of 120°C before one can observe negative effects of heightened temperatures.[46] Furthermore, the literature shows that use of RF with dermal fillers is safe for treated tissue itself if using RF treatments at normal clinical temperatures up to 65°C, which is far beyond the temperature range achieved during EMFACE therapy. Nevertheless, more studies are needed to rule out any possible doubt, especially studies using human participants treated with different ranges of RF intensity and time exposure as well as using multiple different commercially available dermal fillers.

SUMMARY

The novel EMFACE device was developed for noninvasive face lifting and wrinkle reduction by targeting all facial layers, framework, and facial muscles by simultaneously using Synchronized RF and HIFES technologies. Heating the facial tissue to effective temperatures and HIFES stimulation of only specific facial muscles result in a combined effect that causes textural changes to the skin, smoothing, wrinkle reduction, facial repositioning, and an overall lifting effect. The simultaneous and targeted manner of both technologies yields unique benefits by inducing a synergistic effect in the facial soft tissues that cannot be achieved by using these technologies consecutively or as a stand-alone procedure. It poses no risk to patients who underwent neuromodulator or dermal filler procedures and can be safely and effectively used in patients injected with either of them to deliver satisfactory improvement of overall facial appearance.

CLINICS CARE POINTS

- In a long-time botox using patients, the visible contractions start at a higher intensity and after a longer period of time, however in all the patients, the visible contractions were always achieved

- It is normal to observe asymmetrical contractions, when in doubt please palpate the subject. You can adjust the HIFES intensity for each applicator separately

- This therapy uses the radiofrequency, therefore be aware of patients' hydration

DISCLOSURE

Dr S. Chilukuri is a clinical advisor to BTL Industries Ltd. Nonetheless, no funding for authorship and publication of this article was provided, and the author declares no other conflict of interest related to this article.

REFERENCES

1. Coleman S, Grover R. The anatomy of the aging face: Volume loss and changes in 3-dimensional topography. Aesthetic Surg J 2006;26(1):S4–9.
2. Kavanagh S, Newell J, Hennessy M, et al. Use of a neuromuscular electrical stimulation device for facial muscle toning: a randomized, controlled trial. J Cosmet Dermatol 2012;11(4):261–6.
3. Cotofana S, Lowry N, Devineni A, et al. Can smiling influence the blood flow in the facial vein?—An experimental study. J of Cosmetic Dermatology 2020;19(2):321–7.
4. Whitney ZB, Jain M, Jozsa F, Zito PM. Anatomy, Skin, Superficial Musculoaponeurotic System (SMAS) Fascia. In: StatPearls. StatPearls Publishing; 2022. Available at: http://www.ncbi.nlm.nih.gov/books/NBK519014/. Accessed January 29, 2023.
5. Joshi K, Hohman MH, Seiger E. SMAS Plication Facelift. In: StatPearls. StatPearls Publishing; 2022. Available at: http://www.ncbi.nlm.nih.gov/books/NBK531458/. Accessed January 29, 2023.
6. De Jong R, Hohman MH. Brow Ptosis. In: StatPearls. StatPearls Publishing; 2022. Available at: http://www.ncbi.nlm.nih.gov/books/NBK560762/. Accessed January 29, 2023.
7. Araújo AR de, Soares VPC, Silva FS da, et al. Radiofrequency for the treatment of skin laxity: mith or truth. An Bras Dermatol 2015;90(5):707–21.
8. Swift A, Liew S, Weinkle S, et al. The Facial Aging Process From the "Inside Out.". Aesthetic Surg J 2021;41(10):1107–19.
9. Kim K, Jeon S, Kim JK, et al. Effects of Kyunghee Facial Resistance Program (KFRP) on mechanical and elastic properties of skin. J Dermatol Treat 2016;27(2):191–6.
10. Van Borsel J, De Vos MC, Bastiaansen K, et al. The Effectiveness of Facial Exercises for Facial Rejuvenation. Aesthetic Surg J 2014;34(1):22–7.
11. Sulamanidze MA, Paikidze TG, Sulamanidze GM, et al. Facial Lifting with "APTOS" Threads: Featherlift. Otolaryngol Clin 2005;38(5):1109–17.
12. Schultz E, McCormick KM. Skeletal muscle satellite cells. Rev Physiol Biochem Pharmacol 1994;123:213–57.
13. Kakigi R, Naito H, Ogura Y, et al. Heat stress enhances mTOR signaling after resistance exercise in human skeletal muscle. J Physiol Sci 2011;61(2):131–40.
14. Mauro A. Satellite cell of skeletal muscle fibers. J Biophys Biochem Cytol 1961;9:493–5.
15. Langevin HM, Bouffard NA, Fox JR, et al. Fibroblast cytoskeletal remodeling contributes to connective tissue tension. J Cell Physiol 2011;226(5):1166–75.
16. Goto K, Okuyama R, Sugiyama H, et al. Effects of heat stress and mechanical stretch on protein

expression in cultured skeletal muscle cells. Pflügers Archiv European Journal of Physiology 2003;447(2):247–53.

17. Halaas Y, Duncan D, Bernardy J, et al. Activation of Skeletal Muscle Satellite Cells by a Device Simultaneously Applying High-Intensity Focused Electromagnetic Technology and Novel RF Technology: Fluorescent Microscopy Facilitated Detection of NCAM/CD56. Aesthetic Surg J 2021;41(7):NP939–47.

18. Samuels JB, Katz B, Weiss RA. Radiofrequency Heating and High-Intensity Focused Electromagnetic Treatment Delivered Simultaneously: The First Sham-Controlled Randomized Trial. Plast Reconstr Surg 2022;149(5):893e–900e.

19. DiBernardo B, Chilukuri S, McCoy JD, et al. High-Intensity Focused Electromagnetic Field With Synchronized Radiofrequency Achieves Superior Gluteal Muscle Contouring Than High-Intensity Focused Electromagnetic Field Procedure Alone. Aesthet Surg J Open Forum 2023;5:ojac087.

20. Kinney BM, Bernardy J, Jarošová R. Novel Technology for Facial Muscle Stimulation Combined With Synchronized Radiofrequency Induces Structural Changes in Muscle Tissue: Porcine Histology Study. Aesthet Surg J 2023;43(8):920–7.

21. Wong QYA, Chew FT. Defining skin aging and its risk factors: a systematic review and meta-analysis. Sci Rep 2021;11(1):22075.

22. Tobin DJ. Introduction to skin aging. J Tissue Viability 2017;26(1):37–46.

23. Kent D, Fritz K, Salavastru C, et al. Effect of Synchronized Radiofrequency and Novel Soft Tissue Stimulation: Histological Analysis of Connective Tissue Structural Proteins in Skin. Presented at: American Society for Dermatologic Surgery (ASDS) Annual Meeting 2022. October 6-10, 2022; Denver, CO.

24. Bouazizi A, Zaibi G, Samet M, Kachouri A. Parametric study on the dielectric properties of biological tissues. In: 2015 16th International Conference on Sciences and Techniques of Automatic Control and Computer Engineering (STA). IEEE; 2015:54-57. Available at: https://www.semanticscholar.org/paper/Parametric-study-on-the-dielectric-properties-of-Bouazizi-Zaibi/6514f20152d1d0e47b06ca0eb35b89ebada31e87?utm_source=email.

25. Elsaie ML, Choudhary S, Leiva A, et al. Nonablative Radiofrequency for Skin Rejuvenation. Dermatol Surg 2010;36(5):577–89.

26. Goldberg DJ, Lal K. Histological Analysis of Human Skin after Radiofrequency Synchronized with Facial Muscle Stimulation for Wrinkle and Laxity Treatment. Presented at: American Society for Dermatologic Surgery (ASDS) Annual Meeting 2022. October 6-10, 2022; Denver, CO.

27. Halaas Y, Gentile R. The Interim Results of Novel Approach for Facial Rejuvenation. Presented at: American Academy of Facial Plastic and Reconstructive Surgery (AAFPRS) 2022 Annual Meeting. October 20-23, 2022; Washington, DC.

28. Halaas Y., MD. Muscle Quality Improvement Underlines the Non-invasive Facial Remodeling Induced by a Simultaneous Combination of a Novel Facial Muscle Stimulation Technology with Synchronized Radiofrequency. Presented at: American Academy of Facial Plastic and Reconstructive Surgery 2022. October 19-23, 2022; Washington, DC.

29. Kinney B, Boyd C. Safety and Efficacy of Combined HIFES Tissue Stimulation and Monopolar RF for Facial Remodeling. Presented at: American Academy of Facial Plastic and Reconstructive Surgery 2022. October 19-23, 2022; Washington, DC.

30. Nestor MS, Kleinfelder RE, Pickett A. The Use of Botulinum Neurotoxin Type A in Aesthetics: Key Clinical Postulates. Dermatol Surg 2017;43(Suppl 3):S344–62.

31. Segelke B, Knapp M, Kadkhodayan S, et al. Crystal structure of Clostridium botulinum neurotoxin protease in a product-bound state: Evidence for noncanonical zinc protease activity. Proc Natl Acad Sci U S A 2004;101(18):6888–93.

32. Satriyasa BK. Botulinum toxin (Botox) A for reducing the appearance of facial wrinkles: a literature review of clinical use and pharmacological aspect. Clin Cosmet Investig Dermatol 2019;12:223–8.

33. Santus G, Faletti S, Bordanzi I, et al. Effect of short-term electrical stimulation before and after botulinum toxin injection. J Rehabil Med 2011;43(5):420–3.

34. Adams V. Electromyostimulation to fight atrophy and to build muscle: facts and numbers. J Cachexia Sarcopenia Muscle 2018;9(4):631–4.

35. Vyskočil F, Malomouzh A, Nikolsky E. Non-quantal acetylcholine release at the neuromuscular junction. Physiol Res 2009;763–84.

36. Cameron MH. Physical agents in rehabilitation: from research to practice. 4th edition. UK: Elsevier/Saunders; 2013.

37. Frick CG, Richtsfeld M, Sahani ND, et al. Long-term effects of botulinum toxin on neuromuscular function. Anesthesiology 2007;106(6):1139–46.

38. Alfen NV, Gilhuis HJ, Keijzers JP, et al. Quantitative facial muscle ultrasound: feasibility and reproducibility. Muscle Nerve 2013;48(3):375–80.

39. Chilukuri S. Evaluation of Safety and Efficacy of the BTL-785F Device for Non-Invasive Facial Rejuvenation in Patients Injected With Botulinum Toxin. ClinicalTrials.gov identifier: NCT05524766. Updated September 6, 2022. Available at: https://clinicaltrials.gov/ct2/show/NCT05524766. Accessed November 3, 2022.

40. Carruthers J, Carruthers A, Humphrey S. Introduction to Fillers. Plast Reconstr Surg 2015;136(5 Suppl):120S–31S.

41. Commissioner O of the. Dermal Filler Do's and Don'ts for Wrinkles, Lips and More. FDA. Published online April 2, 2022. Available at: https://www.fda.

gov/consumers/consumer-updates/dermal-filler-dos-and-donts-wrinkles-lips-and-more. Accessed January 30, 2023.

42. England LJ, Tan MH, Shumaker PR, et al. Effects of monopolar radiofrequency treatment over soft-tissue fillers in an animal model. Lasers Surg Med 2005; 37(5):356–65.

43. Shumaker PR, England LJ, Dover JS, et al. Effect of monopolar radiofrequency treatment over soft-tissue fillers in an animal model: part 2. Lasers Surg Med 2006;38(3):211–7.

44. Alam M, Levy R, Pajvani U, et al. Safety of radiofrequency treatment over human skin previously injected with medium-term injectable soft-tissue augmentation materials: a controlled pilot trial. Lasers Surg Med 2006;38(3):205–10.

45. Kim H, Park KY, Choi SY, et al. The efficacy, longevity, and safety of combined radiofrequency treatment and hyaluronic Acid filler for skin rejuvenation. Ann Dermatol 2014;26(4):447–56.

46. Goldman MP, Alster TS, Weiss R. A randomized trial to determine the influence of laser therapy, monopolar radiofrequency treatment, and intense pulsed light therapy administered immediately after hyaluronic acid gel implantation. Dermatol Surg 2007; 33(5):535–42.

Aesthetician Role in Facial Plastic Surgery and Systemic Therapy for Healthy Skin

Anya Costeloe, DO[a,b,c,*], James Newman, MD[a]

KEYWORDS

- Aesthetician • Esthetician • Facial plastic surgery • Skin care • Cosmetic surgery • Nutraceuticals
- Vitamins • Systemic therapy

KEY POINTS

- Aestheticians play an important role in facial plastic surgery offices and are an integral part of the care team.
- Aestheticians may assist in the pre- and post-operative care of surgical patients, as well as perform skin care consultations, superficial peels, microdermabrasion, lymphatic massage, dermaplaning, waxing, semi-permanent make-up and other procedures based on specific state laws.
- Regulations on the scope of practice of aestheticians vary widely across states.
- Nutraceuticals are a growing market and as facial plastic surgeons we must educate ourselves on the research and the science behind them.

INTRODUCTION

Aestheticians play an important role in the facial plastic surgeon's office from skin analysis, treatments, early detection of neoplasms, postoperative care from many of the treatments described in this book. They also survey the holistic traditions and explosive array of cosmeceuticals which are constantly changing and help keep us all informed about what many of our patients perceive as good skin maintenance. While there are some comparative standards for the training and certification of aestheticians, we explore the current spectrum of training via interviews with practices across the United States. We also survey the tools and technologies with which aestheticians are able to help our patients achieve optimal skin maintenance.

With the boom of the aesthetic industry, increased life expectancy and the normalization of receiving aesthetic treatment, procedures, and surgeries, facial plastic surgeons are often struggling to have enough time to fulfill patient needs. Aestheticians can complement a busy facial plastic surgery practice by helping in the pre- and post-operative care of patients as well as with skin care and maintenance appointments.

Per the ASCP (Association of Skin Care Professionals), an aesthetician is a skincare professional who focuses on the health and beauty of the skin.[1] Estheticians often work in spas, salons, and resorts, or are self-employed. They may work with clients of all ages and skin types and may specialize in specific areas, such as acne treatment, anti-aging, or eyelash and eyebrow treatments. The role of an aesthetician is to help clients improve the appearance and health of their skin. However, the specific role of the aesthetician working in facial plastic surgery practice varies from practice to practice and from state to state. Some of this variability is due to differences in state laws regarding the scope of practice of aestheticians.

[a] Premier Plastic Surgery, 1795 El Camino Real Suite 200, Palo Alto, CA 94306, USA; [b] The Maas Clinic;
[c] California Pacific Heights Medical Center
* Corresponding author. 1001 4th Street, Southwest washington, DC 20024
E-mail address: anyacosteloe@gmail.com

Facial Plast Surg Clin N Am 31 (2023) 557–566
https://doi.org/10.1016/j.fsc.2023.05.007

TRAINING AND SCOPE OF PRACTICE

Esthetician training and certification requirements vary greatly by state as shown in **Table 1**. While some states have state-specific exams, many states use the National-Interstate Council on State Boards of Cosmetology (NIC) practical and/or written examination. The National Esthetics Practical Examination consists of a section on scientific concepts and a section on esthetics practice. The esthetics practice of the exam covers cleansing and steaming the face, facial makeup, facial mask, hair removal of the eyebrows, manual extraction of the forehead, massaging the face, setup and client protection and so forth.[1]

There are a handful of states (Washington, Virginia, Utah, District of Columbia) that utilize a two tier aesthetician licensing system. Estheticians are able to obtain additional training and take the National Advanced Esthetics Practical Examination (NCEA) to be designated as a "master aesthetician," and NCEA-certified. This is the highest skin credential available in the United States and means the aesthetician has met the competency standards of the NCEA 1200 hour aesthetician job task analysis.[2] The advanced exam covers additional subjects including manual lymphatic drainage, ultrasonic exfoliation treatment, chemical peels, particle microdermabrasion, facial treatment with LED, electricity and electrical equipment, and body treatments such as dry exfoliation and mud mask.

METHODS

Seven states were chosen to represent various regions of the United States. These included California, District of Columbia, Florida, Michigan, New York, Oregon and Texas. The scope of practice and role of aestheticians within facial plastic surgery practices was surveyed in each state by interviewing aestheticians who were employed in facial plastic surgery practices. A questionnaire was created to determine each aesthetician's scope of practice and role, their training and their approach to specific skin concerns. State cosmetology boards were contacted for information was found on their website to find state-specific regulations on aesthetician's scope of practice, training requirements, license requirements, and any recent changes in legislation.

RESULTS

Training and state regulations on the aesthetician's scope of practice vary widely across the country. California has some of the more restrictive regulations while Texas and Michigan allow aestheticians the ability to operate laser devices. Training requirements and state-specific regulations on the scope of practice of aestheticians are shown in **Tables 1** and **2**.

CALIFORNIA

In California (CA), aestheticians are licensed by the California Board of Barbering and Cosmetology and are not allowed to perform medical procedures or diagnose or treat medical conditions. Aestheticians can be hired by a physician to perform non-medical procedures including facials and skin treatments such as microdermabrasion, as long as it is only affecting the outermost layer of the skin, the stratum corneum. Aestheticians may not use lasers or intense pulsed light devices under any circumstance in the state of CA. They are also not allowed to perform microneedling because it penetrates the skin and in a 2016 update on regulation, microneedling was categorized as a medical treatment.[3,4] The most recent update on regulation regarding esthetician is the California Senate Bill 803 that was passed in January 2022. It decreased the barbering and cosmetology programs to 1,000 hours from 1,500 and 1,600 hours and added dermaplaning to the scope of practice for cosmetologists and aestheticians and eyelash and eyebrow perms to the scope of practice for aestheticians.[5]

Unlike aestheticians, medical assistants are regulated by the Medical Board of California. However, they are considered "unlicensed persons" and therefore, are not permitted to perform diagnostic tasks or duties that are invasive or require patient assessment. Overall, the physician is responsible for the appropriate utilization of the medical assistant. A medical assistant can undergo training and licensing by one of the board-approved organizations (American Association of Medical Assistants, American Medical Certification Association, American Medical Technologists, California Certifying Board of Medical Assistants, Multiskilled Medical Certification Institute, Inc.) or receive training from a physician, podiatrist, physician assistant, nurse practitioner or nurse midwife.

A medical assistant is not permitted to perform invasive cosmetic procedures such as microneedling or dermabrasion. However, with the appropriate training, they are able to draw blood and perform skin tests. According to Cal. Code Regs. tit. 16 § 1366.1, a medical assistant can administer medications by intramuscular, subcutaneous, and intradermal injection, perform skin tests, and perform venipuncture to withdraw blood if they

Table 1
Aesthetician training and prerequisites by state

State	Prerequisites	Training	Renewal	Continuing Education (CEU)	Governing Organization
CA	16 yrs old, 10th grade or equivalent	1000 hrs, written & practical exams	Every 2 yrs, $50	None	California Board of Barbering and Cosmetology
DC	16 yrs old, 10th grade	1500 hrs; 2-tier licensing system: basic esthetician and master esthetician licenses	Every 2 years	6hrs every 2 yrs	DC Board of Barber and Cosmetology
FL	16 yrs old, high school diploma or equivalent	260 hrs, written exam	Every 2 yrs, $55	16 hrs every 2 yrs	Florida Department of Business and Professional Regulation
MI	17 yrs old, 9th grade	400 hrs (6 month apprenticeship)	Every 2 yrs, $48	None	Michigan Department of Licensing & Regulatory Affairs – Cosmetology Department
NY	17 yrs old, Certificate from a physician stating the individual is free from communicable diseases	600 hrs, written & practical exams	Every 4 yrs, $40	None	New York Division of Licensing Services-Esthetics
OR	16 yrs old, 8th grade	250 hrs, 150 hrs in safety & infection control, 100 hrs career development, written & practical exams	Every 2 yrs, $40	None, instructor license: 30 hrs every 36 mo	Oregon Health Authority - Board of Cosmetology
TX	17 yrs old, high school diploma or GED	750 hrs, written & practical exams	Every 2 yrs, $50	Speciality Operator License: 4 department approved hours; Instructor License: 6 hours	Texas Department of Licensing & Regulation - Board of Cosmetology

complete minimum training requirements of ten hours of training in the specific procedure and satisfactory of performance of 10 of these procedures.[6] The training must be supervised by a physician or instructor.

FLORIDA

New regulations passed in 2021 limiting the scope of practice of aestheticians. They can no longer perform any service that perforates the skin or

Table 2
Aesthetician scope of practice by state

State	Lasers	Microneedling	Injectables	Noninvasive Procedures[a]
CA	No	No	No	Yes with additional training
DC	Yes if master esthetician	No (can't penetrate past stratum corneum epidermis)	No	Yes with advanced esthetic training certificate
FL	No	No	No	No
MI	Yes	Yes	Unclear	Yes
NY	Yes	No	No	Yes with additional training
OR	No	No	No	Most with advanced esthetic training certificate
TX	Yes	Yes	Under physician supervision	Yes

[a] i.e. noninvasive body contouring, cryolipolysis, noninvasive ultrasound technology, noninvasive radiofrequency technology.

use FDA-approved medical devices. This includes microneedling, laser, pulsed light, ultrasound skincare, radiation skincare, plasma pen or Hyaluron pen services, injections, permanent makeup, and microblading.[7,8]

NEW YORK

New York is one of the few states where there are no limitations on who can operate a laser.[9] However, a new bill that mandates state-approved training, examinations, and continuing certification by an accredited industry group for laser hair removal technicians was proposed in March 2021 and is currently in assembly.[10] Another bill was recently referred to the House Committee on economic development in January 2023 that would allow aestheticians to perform microneedling after completing a five hour course.[11]

OREGON

Based on the rule passed by the Oregon Board of Cosmetology in 2019, aestheticians are not permitted to perform advanced nonablative esthetics, which is defined as "a procedure that uses a laser or other device registered with the United States Food and Drug Administration (USFDA) for nonablative procedures performed on the skin or hair," without a certificate in advanced esthetics.[12] In 2021, the Oregon Estheticians for Fair Licensing (OEFL) requested to pass a law allowing them to use Mechanical or electrical apparatus, appliance or device which do not "penetrate beyond the epidermis except through natural physiological microdermabrasion." These include galvanic current, high-frequency microcurrents, light-emitting diode therapy, and microdermabrasion. However,

the rulemaking process has been paused at this time.[13]

AESTHETICIAN SURVEY RESULTS

Estheticians were interviewed in five states including California, Florida, Michigan, Oregon, and Texas regarding their role in the plastic surgery practice and results are summarized in **Table 3**. Every aesthetician played a role in the perioperative care of the patient, whether it was preparing them for surgery or partaking in postoperative care or both. The common procedures aestheticians perform and the technologies they use vary by state. Based on our survey the most common procedures were peels in Oregon, Florida, and Michigan, facials in California and lasers in Texas. The most common preoperative procedures aestheticians are performing include skin care evaluation and optimization for surgery. Each aesthetician we spoke with plays an important role in the post-operative care of the patient. This includes facials, skin calming treatments, camouflage make-up or simply providing comfort and reassurance during the post-operative visits. In several states aestheticians are performing lymphatic massage and drainage after facelifts.

The most common skin care concerns aestheticians encounter are acne, hyperpigmentation, and aging skin. Recommending and selling skin care products were done by every aesthetician we interviewed and they stated it was an important part of the skin maintenance plan. Some of the biggest challenges aestheticians face are similar to those faced by facial plastic surgeons such as patients having unrealistic expectations and the desire for instantaneous results. The aestheticians

Table 3
Aesthetician survey responses: scope of practice and common procedures

State	Procedures Performed	Most Common Procedure	Degree of Oversight	Pre-Operative	Post-Operative	Skin Care Products
CA	Lymphatic massage VASER®[a] Shape Diamond Glow® Facial Skin Better Science AlphaRet Peels Sofwave® Coolsculpting® Velashape®	Diamond Glow® Facial	Physicians signs all of treatment sheets & charts	Optimizing skin care routine weeks before surgery	Sees patients 2 weeks post-op, US lymphatic massage for face-lift patients	Alastin, Skin Better Science, Isidin
FL	Facials Peels Skin care consultations	Peels	Physician in facility, physician doesn't sign treatment sheets and charts	Skin care assessment and recommendations	Lymphatic drainage, suture removal, skin calming treatments, hydration treatments	Private label, Obagi, Latisse, Viviscal hair vitamins
MI	Facials Micropeels ErbYag laser Diode laser LHR IPL RF microneedling Ulthera® Thermage® Dermaplane	Peels	Physician doesn't see new patients prior to treatment, refers to physician when concerned, physician signs charts	Start skin maintenance prior to surgery, goal 3 treatment prior to Facelift. RetinA for all patients, bleaching cream if needed	Classical facial 4–6 wks after surgery, lymphatic treatment 4–6 wks after surgery, provides comfort, there to hold their hand and tell them their recovery is normal. Reassurance	SkinceuticalObagi, Private label
NY	Lymphatic drainage Peels Hydrafacial	Facials	Physician in facility	Optimize skin care	Lymphatic drainage	Alastin ZO Skin
OR	Facials Waxing Peels Microdermabrasion Microneedling Skin care consults Makeup post-procedure	Peels	Physicians sign all chart notes and treatment plan	Start on a skin care regimen and perform a microdermabrasion treatment	Hydrating facial and camouflage makeup. Sees post-op patients with physician 2–3 times	PCA Skin, ZO Skin

(continued on next page)

Table 3
(continued)

State	Procedures Performed	Most Common Procedure	Degree of Oversight	Pre-Operative	Post-Operative	Skin Care Products
TX	Lasers: fractionated CO2, Cutera XLV® RF microneedling Peels Coolsculpting® TrueFlex® Visia® skin analysis	Laser resurfacing	Physician in facility Physician doesn't sign notes	N/A	Scar treatment	Skinceuticals, Alastin, EltaMD, Skinmedica

Abbreviations: IPL, intense pulsed light; LHR, laser hair removal; RF, radiofrequency.
[a] VASER® shape uses massage therapy and ultrasound technology to smooth and contour different body areas.

we surveyed listed these as well as managing acne and melasma as the most challenging aspects of their job.

DISCUSSION

Aestheticians have become a vital part of many plastic surgery practices and play a unique and important role in the care team. Having non-surgical treatment options can attract patients who are not ready for surgery or complement surgical procedures. New technologies, including lasers, intense pulsed light (IPL), radiofrequency, ultrasound, and other technologies and injectables, are flooding the market and are being used to tighten and resurface skin, decrease pigment, and stimulate collagen production. Skin care is an important part of preparing patients for these procedures as well as in the post-procedure phase.

Skin care consultations are an important part of the aesthetician's job and are a way to bring patients into the practice. In several of the practices we surveyed, aestheticians are using the Visia Skin Analysis (Canfield) to perform skin care consultations with patients as well as track patient progress after undergoing treatment and starting new skin care products. This device uses cross-polarized and UV lighting to quantify sun damage, wrinkles, uneven skin texture, and inflammation. It is also a useful tool for taking before and after photos with controlled head position and lighting.

In a 2004 publication on incorporating skin care into facial plastic surgery practice, laser hair reduction was listed under the services provided by an aesthetician.[14] However, the legislation and regulations around lasers and laser hair removal vary state by state and in the majority of states this is out of the scope of practice of an esthetician.[15] We recommend reaching out to specific medical boards and cosmetology boards to determine specific state regulations.

In most states aestheticians cannot operate lasers, however, aestheticians can play an important role in pre- and post-laser resurfacing treatment of patients, they can see the patient in the immediate post-treatment stage and make sure the patient is using the correct products and sun protection for optimal recovery.

Skin care products are another important component of the non-surgical side of plastic surgery practices. The global skincare market size is growing rapidly and is expected to reach USD 145.82 billion by 2028.[16] A 2020 retrospective study found that more patients who bought skincare products went on to purchase nonsurgical treatments than those who did not buy skin care products.[17] Therefore, being able to offer comprehensive skin care along with products keeps patients happy and introduces them to nonsurgical technology. It justifies and helps sustain investments in non-surgical technologies such as radiofrequency microneedling, intense pulsed light, non-ablative lasers, and electromagnetic muscle toning devices for facial plastic surgery practices and an aesthetician can play an important role here.

NUTRACEUTICALS AND SYSTEMIC SUPPLEMENTS TO PROMOTE HEALTHY SKIN

It is often said that true beauty comes from within. The term nutraceutical was first used in 1989 by Stephen DeFelice, founder and chairman of the Foundation for Innovation in Medicine (FIM), Cranford, New Jersey[18] and came from combining "pharmaceutical" and "nutrition." The Oxford English Dictionary defines nutraceutical as "a foodstuff, food additive, or dietary supplement that has beneficial physiological effects but is not essential to the diet. Also called functional food."[19] The US Nutraceutical Research and Education Act presented to the House of Representatives in the first session of the 106th Congress of 1999–2000 defined nutraceutical as "a dietary supplement, food or medical food … that (1) has a benefit which prevents or reduces the risk of a disease or health condition, including the management of a disease or health condition or the improvement of health; and (2) is safe for human consumption in the quantity, and with the frequency required to realize such properties."[20]

Popularity and use of nutraceuticals and over the counter supplements continues to increase and they are found on the shelf next to skin care items in many facial plastic surgery practices. They can be used before and after surgery to enhance healing or they can be used in combination with non-surgical procedures or independently. Market research by Variant Market Research, Pune, India shows that the nutraceutical industry has been growing at a Compound Annual Growth Rate (CAGR) of 7.2% from 2016 to 2024 and will reach $340 billion by 2024.[21]

Nutraceuticals can be categorized into groups based on the structural class of the main active ingredient. Collagen falls into the category of bioactive peptides. Collagen type I and III is produced by dermal fibroblasts and provide the amino acid building blocks for hair, skin, nails, and bone.[22] Collagen breakdown increases with aging and sun exposure and collagen and elastin decrease with age, therefore, collagen supplementation is a topic of interest in the skin care and cosmetic industry. It has been shown that due to its large molecular weight (130–300 kDa), collagen does not penetrate the epidermis and topical application doesn't provide skin benefits, therefore, oral supplementation with collagen peptides is being studied.[23] Hydrolyzed collagen is made from gelatin and consists of small peptides with low molecular weight and is preferred for oral supplementation because it is rapidly absorbed in the digestive tract. Ingested hydrolyzed collagen is metabolized into small di- or tripeptides and found in the bloodstream two hours after ingestion. One of the dipeptides, proline-hydroxyproline, has been shown to increase cell proliferation (1.5-fold) and hyaluronic acid synthesis (3.8-fold) at a dose of 200 nmol/mL in cultured human dermal fibroblasts.[24]

A study was done in rats looked at 14 C-labeled proline and hydroxyproline in low molecular weight collagen hydrolysate to determine the distribution of ingested collagen in various organs and tissues. They found that the radioactivity in skin at 14 days after ingestion was still elevated at 70% of that six hours after ingestion. By hydrolyzing the skin of the rats, 14 days after ingestion, and analyzing it with thin-layer chromatography, they found that the proline and hydroxyproline were incorporated into the skin. This signifies that orally supplemented collagen hydrolysate can be used for the synthesis of proteins in skin in rats.[25]

The source of collagen is an important factor to consider in oral collagen supplements. Collagen has been derived from bovine, porcine, vegetable, human, marine, and synthetic sources for use in the cosmetic and skin care industry. Marine collagen has been shown to be more easily absorbed than animal collagen, have a lower molecular weight and less biological contaminants.[26]

There have been multiple human clinical trials investigating the benefits of collagen supplementations for skin and anti-aging. A randomized, controlled single-center study with 52 female participants compared daily ingestion of collagen to maltodextrin on skin moisture, elasticity and wrinkle depth. Skin moisture was measured with a corneometer, skin elasticity was measured with a cutometer, and wrinkle depth was analyzed with 3D imaging. They saw an increase in skin moisture index (50.0 $\pm$ 8.7 at T0 and increased to 55.1 $\pm$ 7.8 and 56.8 $\pm$ 8.2 following 28 and

Table 4
Common nutraceuticals and their ingredients

	Nutrafol®	Viviscal®	Skinade®
Vitamins	A, C, D, E, biotin	C, niacin, biotin	C, B-Complex (riboflavin, niacin, biotin, folate, B12)
Minerals	Iodine, zinc, selenium	Calcium, iron, zinc	MSM
Bioactive peptides	Hydrolyzed marine collagen type I & III[a]	AminoMar Marine Complex 536 mg	Hydrolyzed marine collagen 7000 mg
Amino Acids	L-lysine L-methionine L-cysteine		L-lysine
Carotenoid	Astaxanthin		
Bioactive botanical extracts	Organic gelatinized maca root Saw palmetto fruit CO2 extract Ashwagandha extract Liposomal curcumin extract Full-spectrum palm extract Horsetail extract Japanese knotweed root extract (50% resveratrol) Black pepper fruit extract (95% piperine) Capsicum extract	Horsetail extract Millet seed extract	Flaxseed
Polyunsaturated fatty acids			Omega 3 & 6

Abbreviation: MSM, methylsulfonylmethane.
[a] Exact dose unclear as it is listed as an ingredient of the 1875 mg Synergen Complex® Plus.

56 days of treatment (p < 0.01).), mean skin elasticity index (0.604 ± 0.1 at T0 and increased to 0.630 ± 0.1 and 0.651 ± 0.1 following 28 and 56 days of treatment (p < 0.01)), and wrinkle depth (T0 was 0.096 ± 0.01; at T28 and T56, the mean wrinkle depth was 0.092 ± 0.02 and 0.089 ± 0.02, respectively (p < 0.01)).[27]

A double-blind, randomized, placebo-controlled clinical trial was done with n = 120 where 60 subjects were in the control group and took a placebo and 60 subjects received an oral supplement containing collagen type I (5,000 mg), with a molecular weight of 0.3–8 kDa, hyaluronic acid, borage oil and N-acetylglucosamine, vitamins and a blend of antioxidants. The researchers looked at skin elasticity (expressed as Young's elasticity modulus) and skin architecture (histological analysis of biopsies taken in 2 patients) as well as patient satisfaction through questionnaires at day 0 and day 90. They saw a 7.5% increase in skin elasticity in the group receiving the supplement compared to −5% decrease in the control group.[28]

Other types of nutraceuticals include bioactive polysaccharides (glycosaminoglycans), bioactive botanical extracts, carotenoids, vitamins, Coenzyme Q10 (CoQ10), and polyunsaturated fatty acids. Botanical extracts contain polyphenols, which can be further broken down into lignans, flavonoids, flavanols, flavones, flavanones, isflavones, anthrocyanidines, and stilebenes.[29]

Novel formulations are combining the various forms of nutraceuticals to create systemic supplements to promote healthy skin and/or hair (**Table 4**). Skinade® is a skin supplement which includes marine collagen, MSM, vitamin C, l-lysine, flaxseed and vitamin B complex.[30] Nutrafol® and Viviscal® are both hair supplements that have grown in popularity and can be found on the shelves at some facial plastic surgery practices next to skin care products. Nutrafol® contains vitamins A, C, D, and E, biotin, iodine, zinc, selenium and 1875 mg "Synergen Complex® plus" which contains organic gelatinized maca root, saw palmetto fruit CO_2 extract (>45% fatty acids), hydrolyzed marine collagen type I & III, Sensoril® ashwagandha root and leaf extract (10% withanolides), liposomal curcumin (rhizome) extract (>45% curcuminoids), full spectrum palm extract (20% tocotrienol/tocopherol complex), astaxanthin and 480 mg "Nutrafol® Blend" which contains l-lysine, l-methionine, l-cysteine, horsetail extract, Japanese knotweed root extract (50% resveratrol), black pepper fruit extract (95% piperine), capsicum extract (2% capsaicinoids). Viviscal® contains vitamin C, niacin, biotin, calcium, iron, zinc, AminoMar Marine Complex, horsetail extract, and millet seed extract.

SUMMARY

Overall, multiple small studies suggest that nutraceuticals can provide clinically significant benefits for skin and hair, but further research is needed to establish a cause-effect relationship between the ingredients and the beneficial effects for the skin. Current human clinical trials using nutraceuticals often have a low number of subjects. The studies also vary widely in doses of active ingredients and bioavailability is frequently not mentioned. Importantly, caution must be taken when recommending supplements as large doses of some ingredients can be toxic. The facial plastic surgeon must be aware of the importance of choosing nutrients that are well-researched at a dose proven to be effective when recommending nutraceuticals to aesthetic patients.

CLINICS CARE POINTS

- Small studies have shown that nutraceuticals can provide clinically significant benefits for skin and hair, but further research is needed to establish a cause-effect relationship between the ingredients and the beneficial effects.

- Having non-surgical treatment options such as lasers, intense pulsed light (IPL), radiofrequency, ultrasound and other technologies and injectables can attract patients who are not ready for surgery or can complement surgical procedures.

REFERENCES

1. Associated Skin Care Professionals. Associated Skin Care Professionals. http://www.ascpskincare.com. Accessed March 30, 2023.
2. National Certification for Estheticians. NCEA History. https://nceacertified.org/ncea-national-esthetician-association-history/. Accessed March 31, 2023.
3. American Med Spa Association. How Microneedling Is Regulated. https://americanmedspa.org/blog/how-microneedling-is-regulated. Accessed January 29, 2023.
4. Department of Health and Human Services. Classification of the Microneedling Device for Aesthetic Use. Federal Registrar. 2018. Available at: https://www.federalregister.gov/documents/2018/06/08/2018-12335/medical-devices-general-and-plastic-surgery-devices-classification-of-the-microneedling-device-for.

5. American Med Spa Association. American Med Spa Association. SB 803 Barbering and cosmetology., 2021. (testimony of California Legislature).

6. Medical Board of California. Medical Assistants. Medical Board of California. Published 2022. https://www.mbc.ca.gov/Licensing/Physicians-and-Surgeons/Practice-Information/Medical-Assistants.aspx. Accessed January 29, 2023.

7. Pham T., Kemper A., Kemper P., FLORIDA BOARD OF COSMETOLOGY. Published online 2021. Available at: http://www.myfloridalicense.com/dbpr/pro/cosmo/documents/cosmo_minutes_1021.pdf.

8. Pham T., Kemper A., Kemper P., Minutes florida board of cosmetology embassy suites 202 north tamiami trail sarasota, FL 34236. Published online 2021. Available at: http://www.myfloridalicense.com/dbpr/pro/cosmo/documents/cosmo_minutes_1021.pdf.

9. DiGiorgio CM, Avram MM. Laws and regulations of laser operation in the United States. Lasers Surg Med 2018;50(4):272–9.

10. STATE OF NEW YORK IN ASSEMBLY.; 2021.

11. NY State Assembly Bill A2548. https://www.nysenate.gov/legislation/bills/2023/A2548. Accessed March 31, 2023.

12. Oregon Secretary of State Administrative Rules. https://secure.sos.state.or.us/oard/viewSingleRule.action?ruleVrsnRsn=264932. Accessed March 31, 2023.

13. Oregon Health Authority. Oregon Health Authority: HLO News Details: Health Licensing Office: State of Oregon. https://www.oregon.gov/oha/PH/HLO/Pages/News-Details.aspx?View=%7B84858868-A97E-409A-8B8B-ABB77E97CF25%7D&SelectedID=125. Accessed March 31, 2023.

14. TerKonda RP. Incorporating skin care into a facial plastic surgery practice. Minimally Invasive Office-Based Procedures 2004;20(1):3–9.

15. Alam M. Who is qualified to perform laser surgery and in what setting? Semin Plast Surg 2007;21(3):193–200.

16. Skincare Market Share, Growth Industry Trends Analysis. Fortune Business Insights. Published August 2021. https://www.fortunebusinessinsights.com/skin-care-market-102544. Accessed January 22, 2023.

17. Austin R.E., Ahmad J. and Lista F., The impact of skin care product sales in an aesthetic plastic surgery practice. Aesthet Surg J, 40(3), 2020, 330-334.

18. Brower V. Nutraceuticals: Poised for a healthy slice of the healthcare market? Nat Biotechnol 1998;16(8):728–31.

19. Nutraceutical: Oxford English Dictionary. Published December 2022. https://www.oed.com/. Accessed April 1, 2023.

20. Aronson JK. Defining 'nutraceuticals': neither nutritious nor pharmaceutical. Br J Clin Pharmacol 2017;83(1):8–19.

21. Variant Market Research. Nutraceuticals Market Global Scenario, Market Size,Trend and Forecast, 2015-2024. https://www.variantmarketresearch.com/report-categories/food-beverages/nutraceuticals-market/. Accessed March 31, 2023.

22. Cole MA, Quan T, Voorhees JJ, et al. Extracellular matrix regulation of fibroblast function: redefining our perspective on skin aging. J Cell Commun Signal 2018;12(1):35–43.

23. Bos JD, Meinardi MMHM. The 500 Dalton rule for the skin penetration of chemical compounds and drugs. Exp Dermatol 2000;9:165–9. Available at: http://chemfinder.

24. Ohara H, Ichikaya S, Matsumoto H, et al. Collagen-derived dipeptide, proline-hydroxyproline, stimulates cell proliferation and hyaluronic acid synthesis in cultured human dermal fibroblasts. J Dermatol 2010;37(4):330–8.

25. Watanabe-Kamiyama M, Shimizu M, Kamiyama S, et al. Absorption and effectiveness of orally administered low molecular weight collagen hydrolysate in rats. J Agric Food Chem 2010;58(2):835–41.

26. Avila Rodríguez MI, Rodríguez Barroso LG, Sánchez ML. Collagen: a review on its sources and potential cosmetic applications. J Cosmet Dermatol 2018;17(1):20–6.

27. Bianchi FM, Angelinetta C, Rizzi G, et al. Evaluation of the efficacy of a hydrolyzed collagen supplement for improving skin moisturization, smoothness, and wrinkles. J Clin Aesthet Dermatol 2022;15(3):48–52.

28. Genovese L, Corbo A, Sibilla S. An insight into the changes in skin texture and properties following dietary intervention with a nutricosmeceutical containing a blend of collagen bioactive peptides and antioxidants. Skin Pharmacol Physiol 2017;30(3):146–58.

29. Pérez-Sánchez A, Barrajón-Catalán E, Herranz-López M, et al. Nutraceuticals for skin care: a comprehensive review of human clinical studies. Nutrients 2018;10(4):403.

30. Anderson KL. Clinical Evidence of the Anti-Aging Effects of a Collagen Peptide Nutraceutical Drink on the Skin. Published online 2020.

UNITED STATES POSTAL SERVICE ®
Statement of Ownership, Management, and Circulation
(All Periodicals Publications Except Requester Publications)

1. Publication Title	2. Publication Number		3. Filing Date
FACIAL PLASTIC SURGERY CLINICS OF NORTH AMERICA	013 – 122		9/18/2023

4. Issue Frequency	5. Number of Issues Published Annually	6. Annual Subscription Price
FEB, MAY, AUG, NOV	4	$428.00

7. Complete Mailing Address of Known Office of Publication (Not printer) (Street, city, county, state, and ZIP+4®)

ELSEVIER INC.
230 Park Avenue, Suite 800
New York, NY 10169

Contact Person: Malathi SAmayan
Telephone (Include area code): 91-44-4299-4507

8. Complete Mailing Address of Headquarters or General Business Office of Publisher (Not printer)

ELSEVIER INC.
230 Park Avenue, Suite 800
New York, NY 10169

9. Full Names and Complete Mailing Addresses of Publisher, Editor, and Managing Editor (Do not leave blank)

Publisher (Name and complete mailing address)

Dolores Meloni, ELSEVIER INC.
1600 JOHN F KENNEDY BLVD. SUITE 1600
PHILADELPHIA, PA 19103-2899

Editor (Name and complete mailing address)

Stacy Eastman ELSEVIER INC.
1600 JOHN F KENNEDY BLVD. SUITE 1600
PHILADELPHIA, PA 19103-2899

Managing Editor (Name and complete mailing address)

PATRICK MANLEY, ELSEVIER INC.
1600 JOHN F KENNEDY BLVD. SUITE 1600
PHILADELPHIA, PA 19103-2899

10. Owner (Do not leave blank. If the publication is owned by a corporation, give the name and address of the corporation immediately followed by the names and addresses of all stockholders owning or holding 1 percent or more of the total amount of stock. If not owned by a corporation, give the names and addresses of the individual owners. If owned by a partnership or other unincorporated firm, give its name and address as well as those of each individual owner. If the publication is published by a nonprofit organization, give its name and address.)

Full Name	Complete Mailing Address
WHOLLY OWNED SUBSIDIARY OF REED/ELSEVIER, US HOLDINGS	1600 JOHN F KENNEDY BLVD. SUITE 1600 PHILADELPHIA, PA 19103-2899

11. Known Bondholders, Mortgagees, and Other Security Holders Owning or Holding 1 Percent or More of Total Amount of Bonds, Mortgages, or Other Securities. If none, check box ▶ ☐ None

Full Name	Complete Mailing Address
N/A	

12. Tax Status (For completion by nonprofit organizations authorized to mail at nonprofit rates) (Check one)
The purpose, function, and nonprofit status of this organization and the exempt status for federal income tax purposes:
☒ Has Not Changed During Preceding 12 Months
☐ Has Changed During Preceding 12 Months (Publisher must submit explanation of change with this statement)

PS Form **3526**, July 2014 (Page 1 of 4 (see instructions page 4)) PSN 7530-01-000-9931 PRIVACY NOTICE: See our privacy policy on www.usps.com

---

13. Publication Title	14. Issue Date for Circulation Data Below
FACIAL PLASTIC SURGERY CLINICS OF NORTH AMERICA	AUGUST 2023

15. Extent and Nature of Circulation		Average No. Copies Each Issue During Preceding 12 Months	No. Copies of Single Issue Published Nearest to Filing Date
a. Total Number of Copies (Net press run)		175	171
b. Paid Circulation (By Mail and Outside the Mail)	(1) Mailed Outside-County Paid Subscriptions Stated on PS Form 3541 (Include paid distribution above nominal rate, advertiser's proof copies, and exchange copies)	118	123
	(2) Mailed In-County Paid Subscriptions Stated on PS Form 3541 (Include paid distribution above nominal rate, advertiser's proof copies, and exchange copies)	0	0
	(3) Paid Distribution Outside the Mails Including Sales Through Dealers and Carriers, Street Vendors, Counter Sales, and Other Paid Distribution Outside USPS®	27	21
	(4) Paid Distribution by Other Classes of Mail Through the USPS (e.g. First-Class Mail®)	9	6
c. Total Paid Distribution (Sum of 15b (1), (2), (3), and (4)) ▶		154	150
d. Free or Nominal Rate Distribution (By Mail and Outside the Mail)	(1) Free or Nominal Rate Outside-County Copies included on PS Form 3541	20	20
	(2) Free or Nominal Rate In-County Copies Included on PS Form 3541	0	0
	(3) Free or Nominal Rate Copies Mailed at Other Classes Through the USPS (e.g. First-Class Mail)	0	0
	(4) Free or Nominal Rate Distribution Outside the Mail (Carriers or other means)	1	1
e. Total Free or Nominal Rate Distribution (Sum of 15d (1), (2), (3) and (4)) ▶		21	21
f. Total Distribution (Sum of 15c and 15e) ▶		175	171
g. Copies not Distributed (See Instructions to Publishers #4 (page 43)) ▶		0	0
h. Total (Sum of 15f and g) ▶		175	171
i. Percent Paid (15c divided by 15f times 100) ▶		87.99%	87.72%

* If you are claiming electronic copies, go to line 16 on page 3. If you are not claiming electronic copies, skip to line 17 on page 3.

PS Form **3526**, July 2014 (Page 2 of 4)

16. Electronic Copy Circulation	Average No. Copies Each Issue During Preceding 12 Months	No. Copies of Single Issue Published Nearest to Filing Date
a. Paid Electronic Copies ▶		
b. Total Paid Print Copies (Line 15c) + Paid Electronic Copies (Line 16a) ▶		
c. Total Print Distribution (Line 15f) + Paid Electronic Copies (Line 16a) ▶		
d. Percent Paid (Both Print & Electronic Copies) (16b divided by 16c × 100) ▶		

☒ I certify that 50% of all my distributed copies (electronic and print) are paid above a nominal price.

17. Publication of Statement of Ownership

☒ If the publication is a general publication, publication of this statement is required. Will be printed in the NOVEMBER 2023 issue of this publication. ☐ Publication not required.

18. Signature and Title of Editor, Publisher, Business Manager, or Owner	Date
Malathi Samayan - Distribution Controller *Malathi Samayan*	9/18/2023

I certify that all information furnished on this form is true and complete. I understand that anyone who furnishes false or misleading information on this form or who omits material or information requested on the form may be subject to criminal sanctions (including fines and imprisonment) and/or civil sanctions (including civil penalties).

PS Form **3526**, July 2014 (Page 3 of 4) PRIVACY NOTICE: See our privacy policy on www.usps.com

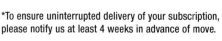

Printed and bound by CPI Group (UK) Ltd, Croydon, CR0 4YY

08/05/2025

01864749-0016

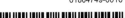